CANDIDA M. ALLERGY

G000125185

The Way Back to Good Health
An A-Z
By Jo Hampton

Copyright Jo Hampton
1st Edition 1993
Reprinted in 1997
Revised edition 2001

ISBN 0-9521544-4-7

Published by R.F.Hampton
KINGSTON HOUSE PUBLISHING,
13, Glenwood Gardens, Hope Corner Lane,
Taunton, Somerset. TA2 7PA Tel/Fax 01823 35 11 08
E:Mail johampton@earthdust.freeserve.co.uk

Printed in the UK
by
*DACOSTA PRINT
1A Mildmay Avenue,
London N1 4RS
(020 7354 6200)*

Jo Hampton has been a practising Alternative and Complimentary Health Consultant for many years. Since early in 1980 she has specialized in immuno-deficiency conditions. Her articles have been published in a number of periodicals and she has been quoted as an authority by other authors in works dealing with Candida, M.E. and allergies. She has lectured extensively. Jo is married with 2 daughters and 4 grandchildren.

This was her first book. Since the first edition in 1993 it has been reprinted twice. This revised edition has been carefully updated to include advances made and to reflect the added experience Jo has acquired since that time.

Dedicated to all those who gave me the encouragement to write this book, and to all who will regain good health by following the instructions set out herein.

Other books by this author are:-

Cooking for Candida
(Diet Plans and Recipes with Vegetarian options)
I.S.B.N. 0-9521544-1-2

The Arthritis Cookbook and Drug Free Treatment Plan
(With vegetarian options)
I.S.B.N. 0-9521544-2-0

" ....within 2 weeks of starting the treatment I felt 100 times better......"

Pregnant Candida sufferer, Reigate, Sussex.

"....my daughter has improved greatly since following the diet programme along with the right supplements..."

Grateful Mother, Glasgow.

"....I have suffered mouth ulcers for 25 years.... after only 2 months I can eat, sleep, taste, talk, swallow, (and kiss) without pain. Imagine my relief!....."

Allergy sufferer, Harlow, Middlesex.

"...at my worst, I wanted my bowel removed, it hurt so much. I don't wake up in the night in agony anymore, thanks to your advice....."

Mother of 6, Whitstable, Kent.

" .....It actually worked.... I even have enough energy to party, AND DANCE. Thanks..."

18 year old M.E. sufferer, Basildon, Essex.

"....I have never felt better in my life. My capacity to cope with people and pressures is greater than it has ever been. I am indebted to you...."

Chartered Accountant with Allergies.

CONTENTS

5

INTRODUCTION - my own experience

I opened my eyes to a bedroom filled with late summer sunlight. Slowly my hand reached down and touched my abdomen. My mind thrilled, awake to the certain knowledge that I was pregnant, and oh! so happy to be.

Gradually I became aware of my child's father, still sleeping blissfully beside me. Why wasn't he at work? Then I realized, it was a public holiday. He was mine all day! I reached out and traced a soft line down his relaxed face. His blue eyes flickered open, focusing on me. A grin spread from them to his mouth, letting me know I was loved. He reached out for me, and I snuggled contentedly into the circle of his arms. Our lips met, I felt myself warm to his touch. Then it happened..... My head exploded, pain shot through me. More intense pain than I had ever dreamed possible. I felt sick and vomited. Ben, my husband said, "What's the matter? " "I don't know," I replied, "Perhaps I am losing the baby. Get me something to settle my stomach and a pain killer." He hurried to the bathroom cabinet, returning with them, plus a glass of water. Looking worried, he stood by the bed and held the glass out to me. I tried to take it, but my arm wouldn't move. I endeavoured to sit up, but my body refused to obey. Now I was frightened, this was no miscarriage.

"Phone the doctor," I said, realizing my mouth was having difficulty framing the words. Our doctor, one of the old school who knew the family by name and was interested in us as people, was with us within fifteen minutes. Before half an hour had passed I was in an ambulance, on my way to the nearest hospital with a neurosurgical unit. I had suffered a cerebral haemorrhage... That day was to change my life.

By the time I reached hospital, I was totally paralysed down the left side. I had lost my speech, and my sight was severely restricted. The hospital staff were efficient and morphine was given to ease the pain. Tubes were inserted into my nose and throat, to prevent me choking on my own vomit. I was hooked up to a glucose drip and a host of other indignities were perpetrated on my inert, unsuspecting, 27 year old body. Heavy sedation was necessary to keep me still until my condition stabilized then an operation was performed to reduce the bleeding from the aneurysm in my head. They saved my life, and I am grateful.

I was released from hospital five weeks later, extremely stiff, and bloated as a consequence of the drugs and the operation, but no longer paralysed. However the whole of the left side of my body lacked co-ordination and I had difficulty finding words, although my mind knew them. I would stop, mid-sentence, searching for the right word to express my thought, knowing it was in my brain somewhere, but failing to summon it to my tongue. I felt old and slow. Every reaction was delayed. My body didn't feel as though it belonged to me. Everything ached and creaked. But joy of joys! *I WAS STILL PREGNANT.*

The doctors were worried that my head would go off bang again if I was allowed to have a normal birth so it was decided I should go straight to hospital at the first sign of labour and be delivered by caesarean section. I knew of no alternative and trusted them implicitly. I was assured it would be much less painful than a natural birth. I need worry about nothing.

So on February 21st 1967 my second child was lifted from a gaping hole in my abdomen, whilst I was strapped by the wrists and ankles to a tilted operating table, under heavy anaesthetic.

I awoke several hours later to indescribable back pain and a tightness in my lungs. It was impossible to cough, it hurt too much so I contented myself with a wheeze. The trouble in my lungs turned out to be an allergic reaction to the anaesthetic.

They brought my beautiful daughter for me to hold, but the pain that racked my body made it impossible for me to hold her long enough to feed her, which had been my strong desire and firm resolve. I did however, satisfy myself she was whole. The trauma we had both experienced whilst she was in the womb had not physically damaged her. Everything was there.

Three weeks later Ben collected me along with his new baby daughter, from the hospital. We went home joyous to be together again

9

with our long awaited addition to the family.

The doctors at the hospital assured me the continuous pain I was experiencing was all quite normal, and it would go with time. They gave me some pain killers to tide me over. The pills were strong and made me sleepy, but without them, lifting the baby and everyday chores were impossible.

Our baby was about six weeks old when I suddenly developed a lump in my neck, close to the scar left by the surgery performed for the cerebral haemorrhage. It was extremely painful and prevented me moving my head. When my doctor saw it he sent me immediately to a small local hospital.

Another anaesthetic was administered and surgery was executed to remove the lump. It was all done in a matter of hours. I was detained in hospital for a week under observation. I never met the surgeon who did the operation, but when his young assistant did the ward rounds, I asked him what had been found. He muttered something about the time when we were fishes, and evolution, then said that my gills had become infected. He looked so uncomfortable. It was obviously a 'cock and bull' story. I told him I was not a fool and I wanted to be told the truth. He refused to meet my gaze and said he was not at liberty to tell me and that I should ask my doctor when I went home.......
I did, and this is how the conversation went.....

Me:- "Well what was it?"
Dr:- "Nothing to worry about."
Me:- "But I want to know what it was."
Dr:- "I can't tell you."
Me:- "I have a right to know. After all it is my body."
Dr:- "I can't tell you! But I'll tell you a story...... My dad was a surgeon, and he always made a point of wearing boots a size too large in the operating theatre when he operated, so that if, when he opened up the patient, he found something a previous surgeon had left behind, he could drop it into his boot and avoid a fuss."
Me:- "So you are telling me something was left behind from the other operation?"
Dr:- "No, I didn't say that. Lets not talk anymore. You are all right now

and there are people waiting outside."

When I returned home, I thought seriously about consulting a solicitor, but I had sustained three operations in less than a year and felt too ill to fight.... So I let it go. (When we moved in 1990, I had access to my case notes. All mention of the last operation had been removed from my file.)

I began to doubt the medical profession, but at the time, I knew no alternative but to take their advice.

After that last operation, as the baby grew and became heavier, I was in more and more pain. I went to the doctor repeatedly seeking relief. At one stage he sent me to hospital outpatients for physiotherapy. First I was given traction. Next heat treatment, one thing after another, but nothing made any difference. Finally I was sent for x-rays on my spine. The consultant diagnosed arthritis. By this time I had begun to vomit after practically every meal, my hair was falling out, my nails refused to grow, and what was left of them cracked and split.

My bowels were in a mess. Either I would not go for days, or I would have diarrhoea. My feet were so painful I could hardly bear my weight on them and my joints were so stiff I moved like an eighty year old. Ben was having to lift me out of bed each morning and help me to dress. All the time I was popping more and more pain killers just to make it through the day.

I went yet again to the doctor, determined to get some real help this time. He said I was going to have to learn to live with it. "In fact" he said, "I estimate that you will probably be in a wheelchair within two years." *"NO I ********WON'T,"* I said, and left his office. *ANGRY. .... I had finally lost all confidence in allopathic medicine's ability to help me.*

My anger translated itself into a strong determination to find a way to help myself back to the good health I had known before the haemorrhage occurred. Of course, I realized there would be some things I could do nothing about, but after all, I wasn't yet 30 years old and a wheelchair was totally unacceptable to me. I began to read.... Anything

11

I could find on alternative and complementary medicine. Cautiously I began trying different therapies. Chiropractic was the first big breakthrough. The highly skilled practitioner whose help I sought, was able to identify and put right the cause of the majority of my neck and back pain. He found two vertebrae misplaced due to the operations I had been subjected to. He gently eased them back into place and within days I was freed from some of the excruciating pain I had experienced for so long.

It wasn't the entire answer though. So I began to read up on nutrition and realized my diet left much to be desired. Immediately I set about changing it. What evolved was a diet high in fibre and whole foods, with as much fresh produce as possible, and nothing with preservatives. I began to feel small changes in my body. My vitality lifted and I was less stiff. Also my bowels improved a bit. I knew I must be on the right track so I began to take vitamin supplements and gained more improvement, but still I knew there was more to it. Now I had more energy and less pain, I decided to take a course in nutrition and one in reflexology. It was at one of these I met a lady who told me about the work of Dr Richard Mackarness. I read his book called "It's Not all in the Mind." In it he described how some foods could make allergic people ill. Suddenly the fact I often had pain, or worsening of symptoms after a meal, held new significance for me.

Was I suffering from allergy?... Had my body become weighed down with chemical overload, due to the allopathic medication I had been subjected to over the years? Could allergy be the real reason for the way I looked and felt? Excited by the prospect of a breakthrough, I bought more reading matter on the subject. One of the books I purchased listed 49 symptoms that could be caused by allergies .... I had 29 of them.

Soon I became aware there was nobody in England at that time, either in orthodox or alternative medicine, who understood allergy. Neither was anyone prepared to train in or treat it.

Money was short in our little family, so the idea of travelling to America to seek help was out of the question. So how could I help myself? In several of the books by Dr. Mackarness, Theron Randolph

M.D. had been mentioned as a clinical ecologist who specialized in treating and writing on the subject of allergy. I sent to America for his books. Also work by Marshall Mandell, M.D. As I read through these books I became positive I had at last identified my problem. Each of the books advocated a five day fast, a total fast on nothing but spring water. After this it was recommended to introduce one food at a time, noting any reactions. This would identify personal allergens. Of course we have kinder methods to identify allergens nowadays but then it was all I knew and I was determined to try. I had only the books to explain what I must do and what might happen. I warned my family, friend's and our family doctor of my intentions. Some said I wouldn't survive without food, others said I would give in and eat after half a day. They didn't know how ill I felt, or my determination to regain my health.

I comforted myself with the thought, if Jesus could last out for 40 days I could surely manage 5.

IT WORKED........ By the fifth day without food I felt so well I decorated a bedroom and laid tiles on our kitchen floor. I really did feel good in my mind as well as my body. Then came the crunch. I had to start eating again, and challenging myself.

The first food I selected to break my fast was, I thought, the least innocuous. Cows milk yoghurt. Within minutes, my whole mouth erupted with herpes simplex blisters. They eventually spread to my nose and chin. Chips came next. No reaction. Good! I had lots because I now realized how hungry I had become. Cautiously, individually I tried a variety of vegetables. All proved fine.

Then came bread. Disaster! Within 20 minutes you would have sworn I had consumed at least half a bottle of whisky. I behaved as though I was well and truly drunk. Ben lovingly carried me, giggling uncontrollably, off to bed, and tucked me up to sleep it off. I dared him to let anyone see me like it as they would never have believed the truth.

My next bad result was when I ate lamb. All the theories about lamb and pears being safe for people with food allergies were proved wrong. After just a few mouthfuls I fell asleep for 4 hours, only waking when my bowels went berserk.

13

Some of the reactions I experienced were truly horrendous, affecting my mind as well as my body. At one stage I remember cowering in a corner like a trapped animal, wild eyed, screaming abuse at my kind, loving, long suffering husband. It testifies to his love that he stayed with me during those terrible times. A lesser mortal would have found solace elsewhere, or maybe had me committed.

I continued in this way, introducing a new food only after I was sure all chance of reaction to the previous one was past. Soon I had established a list of foods that were safe for me to eat. I also made a list of foods to avoid. Then I built my diet around the 'safe' foods.

Time passed and I stuck rigidly to my diet, fearful of the pain and other symptoms returning if I broke my self inflicted rules.

Soon my hair began to shine again, my skin improved, my nails grew and I began to lead a normal life for the first time in years.

People who had known me during the bad times would stop me in the street and ask, "Is it really you? You look so well, so different. What have you done?" I was happy to tell them what I had learned, and soon people began bringing their friends, family and children to see me, asking for my advice on allergies.

It was then I began to realize two things. Firstly, not everyone had my determination and willpower where fasting was concerned, and secondly, I was inadequately equipped to give advice to sick people. So I started studying again. It was about this time when Applied Kinesiology came to my attention. Imagine my delight when I discovered sensitivities to both food and chemicals could be identified without the agony of a 5 day fast / challenge process.

I became convinced there had to be a clinical explanation for why one person reacted whilst another didn't. I was still looking for an underlying *CAUSE.* For a long time the answer escaped me - until the works of C. Orion Truss M.D. (The Missing Diagnosis) and William Crook M.D. (The Yeast Connection) came into my hands. Both doctors identified the parasite Candida albicans as being responsible for breaking down immune system responses.

14

At once, I realized if allergies were to be overcome and normal immune system function regained, the parasite would have to be eliminated and immunity restored. Immuno deficiency was the true missing link.

However, I was always aware that, although I had gained remission from most of my symptoms, this was only true whilst I avoided my known allergens. If I ate something I shouldn't, or came into contact with certain chemicals, my symptoms would reappear. I still hadn't found the entire answer. There had to be more.

So, starting with myself, I began to treat Candida albicans, developing a treatment programme not only to knock out the Candida, but also to rebuild the immune system. Within 6 months I felt better than at any time in my life. Over a period of time my sensitivities faded, one by one, until I no longer reacted to foods and chemicals as I had done. I felt marvellous! I had found *the way back to health.*

Then I turned my attention to all the people who contacted me for help, not only those with identifiable allergies, but also those with Candida albicans, M.E. and arthritis, in fact many immune deficiency based diseases responded to the carefully balanced regime I recommended. They all made startling improvements as their immune systems were strengthened.

Soon word spread, and I was sending details of my methods everywhere. It wasn't long before people from all over the world began visiting me for consultations. As they applied my advice their health returned.

Over the years people have repeatedly urged me to write down the advice I gave to them, enabling them to resume a normal way of life.

So here it is .... You too can find....

"THE WAY BACK TO HEALTH"

ACCEPTANCE

Often people find it hard to accept Candida albicans as the condition responsible for their many symptoms and the terrible way they feel. They keep hoping they really aren't that bad and if they ignore the symptoms they will eventually go away. Others are too proud to admit to any kind of illness. They view it as a weakness and refuse to concede to the need for help. (This is mostly men, but by no means all).

Doctors are often unable to help. Few people are aware that in five years of medical training, less than five hours is devoted to nutrition and the role of supplements. There is very little recognition of Candida and M.E. by the orthodox medical profession, in spite of the British government giving M.E. official recognition by the N.H.S. in October 1997. Consequently, diagnosis of these allied conditions are often dismissed. The symptoms are then treated individually and the sufferer is sent on a time consuming and tiring round of specialist's waiting rooms.

People with good jobs sometimes delay seeking treatment because they feel themselves to be indispensable. Or for fear they will be replaced if they don't keep up the pace. Both reasons are faulty. If an employee has made themselves truly indispensable (which is very rare) then their employer will have a vested interest in waiting for them to regain their health, encouraging and helping wherever possible, so the sufferer is able to return to duty as soon as possible with added vigour. The second argument fails because, without treatment, their health will continue to deteriorate and eventually they will slow down and stop entirely. The sooner they begin treatment, the less likely they are to lose their job. Remember, Candida can become very serious, even life threatening. The longer it is allowed to ravage the immune system un-untreated, the more long term damage it may cause, possibly doing irreversible damage to major organs and becoming a precursor to M.E.

"So accept your problem and deal with it fast"

Under this heading it would be appropriate to include a word or two more about the acceptance of your problem by the orthodox medical profession. If you don't expect any real help or understanding from them then you will not be disappointed or frustrated when none is forthcoming. What you can expect is an offer of psychiatric advice or drugs. Neither will prove beneficial. In the average doctor's estimation you are suffering from:-

> *A) Your nerves.*
> *B) Stress.*
> *C) Your age.*
> *D) Galloping hypochondria.*

Or in his opinion there is nothing wrong with you at all.

Some years ago, a young woman was led by the hand into my consulting room by her very concerned, loving husband. She could not speak for herself. She just sat, hands crossed over a drab cardigan buttoned up wrongly, hanging her head, unable to take interest in anything going on around her. Her hair was lank, straggling over her shoulders, her stockings twisted about her ankles. I tried addressing questions to her, but to no avail.

Her husband told me she was 35 years old. I had estimated her to be between 48 and 53. He related a story with which I have become all too familiar. She became tired and lethargic after the birth of their fourth child, developing 'flu-type' symptoms. The doctor prescribed antibiotics 'to clear it up.' Her lethargy worsened and she developed pains in her abdomen. Appendicitis was diagnosed. She was admitted to hospital where her appendix was removed. It proved quite healthy. When she woke from the anaesthetic she still had her pain. More exploratory surgery was performed, but nothing found to be physically wrong with her.

By this time, not surprisingly, she was depressed. It was suggested she needed to see a psychiatrist. She agreed but could not be convinced her pain was not of very real physical origin. Her husband was beginning to doubt her by this time, and persuaded her to try the drugs offered to 'cheer her up.' Her condition rapidly deteriorated, until she was admitted to the psychiatric unit of her local hospital. She had been there for six months, when her husband heard about Candida from

17

a friend who had been my client. With her husband's co-operation I worked out a diet and supplement plan for her and weaned her off the drugs she was taking, giving her supplements indicated by her condition. Within days her husband reported improvement. Several months later I walked through the waiting room wondering what all the laughter was about and was met by a vibrant, beautifully dressed young woman who was confidently flirting with my husband. She was very difficult to recognize without her Candida problem.

I include this story because it illustrates, not only the need for sufferers to recognize their symptoms for what they are, but also the terrible consequences to their patients when doctors refuse to acknowledge the existence of these health problems.

Having said that, there are an increasing number of doctors who are informing themselves and recognizing the problem, although they still remain baffled as to how to treat it because all they have in their tool bag is drugs, which only make matters worse for the patient (See N for Nystatin). Just a few doctors are prepared to recommend the patient buys the strong vitamins and bacteria supplements necessary, but as yet they are not fighting the strangle hold on medicine held by the big drug companies who subsidize the training medical students receive. Their training is therefore restrictive and their hands are tied by the establishment.

Try to accept their position. The system ties their hands, but your hands are free......

"You CAN help yourself"

Once you have accepted Candida as the possible cause of your problems, obtain a positive diagnosis from a competent practitioner and start setting yourself right.

(See heading *ADVICE*)

ACCOUNTABILITY

We are all accountable to someone. Be it a husband, wife, child, parents, work associates or just society in general. We owe it to those to whom we are accountable to function well. If our health is impaired and there is something we know we could do to improve it, then we should feel obligated to do so. Not only will family relationships improve and our friendships blossom, but our earning capacity will soar when our concentration and work efficiency is enhanced as our energy levels rise. Good health improves every facet of life, so we should all strive to achieve the optimum available to us. If we are apt to think the supplements required to attain health are too costly, perhaps we should analyse the way we use money available to us. In doing this remember we are not just out to improve our own quality of life but to benefit those around us. They are spared worry and concern about us, also our moaning and complaints about our symptoms. They may also be freed from caring for us and be able to enjoy their own lives more.

So never begrudge money spent on health supplements. Think how much it costs to smoke, drink alcohol, take drugs, buy theatre tickets, videos, beauty products, suntan lotions, expensive holidays, trash reading matter and a host of other unnecessary items.

"Think positive and you will see, buying good health is getting your priorities right."

Good health is the best insurance you can own. When you are healthy you can work. When you work you earn. When you earn you catch up on all the things you go without in order to be well.

I know a lady who went without a new outfit for a wedding, having a crown fitted on her teeth instead. She commented that the crown not only improved her appearance long term, but had also aided her digestion. In her estimation it was the better buy. Another invested in a set of heated rollers to cut hairdressing fees. Spending the savings on supplements. We not only owe it to others to be well, but...

"We owe it to ourselves"

ADVICE - Choosing the right kind

Finding a practitioner can be fraught with problems. Even those displaying *bona fide* qualifications may have earned them years earlier and be out of touch with ecologically related health problems and latest treatments available. Many practitioners may have trained but never actually helped a client through to a satisfactory conclusion. Recommendation is the best. Perhaps someone you know has similar problems. Ask if they are seeing anyone. If they are, enquire whether they are satisfied with their progress, and how long they have been attending.

If their health has improved in a reasonable amount of time, and they speak well of the practitioner, ask for the name and telephone number. Call them. Don't be put off by an answer phone. A good practitioner doesn't always have a receptionist, but will not allow the phone to interrupt a consultation. Think, if you were the client, would you want time from your appointment taken up by casual enquiries? Of course not. You want individual attention. An answer phone may ensure you get it. If a machine answers your call, listen to the message, then call again at the time suggested, or leave your name and number requesting they call you. If you are answered by a receptionist, ask about methods used and fees charged etc. When a good practitioner employs staff, they choose kindly helpful people. However, you do need to be discerning in your choice, or you could end by paying large fees for treatments, consultations and supplements not suited to your needs.

There is a tendency among sick people to become desperate for any kind of help, this may lead them to try several treatments a once. This can cause confusion. One treatment may render another impotent and if you do have some improvement, how will you know which one is working for you? Take one at a time, and give it a chance. You won't get a miracle! It takes nine months for the immune system to develop in the womb therefore you must expect a similar time to repair it when damage has been done. What you can expect are changes in your condition, slow progression back to health and well being. If you seek advice from other sufferers, Make sure they are *positive thinkers.*

Someone who has tried a treatment and gained no benefit from it, could be a person who will not maintain the suggested diet, or repeatedly fails to take the recommended supplements. In a case like that, it is not the treatment that has failed, nor the practitioner, but the client. These people can be very depressing, undermining your confidence and determination. Question them closely to discover why the treatment failed before you reject it.

If possible try to speak personally to the practitioner before you make a firm appointment. You need to be able to understand their 'language.' If you do not understand the way they talk to you, it is very unlikely you will benefit from a consultation. Please remember though, if they are good, they will be busy and unable to spend hour upon hour on the phone.

A good practitioner takes cleanliness seriously, so they will make sure their premises and their person are clean and neat. This does not mean the place has to be full of expensive furnishings, just clean, tidy and well suited to the purpose for which it is used.

Above all, be sure you are able to establish a good relationship with your chosen practitioner. You need to feel comfortable and relaxed with them so you are able to confide your innermost fears, not feel overawed or intimidated by them. View them as a friend who is truly interested in you.

"Be cautious and then be confident"

ALCOHOL

Should a Candida or M.E. sufferer indulge in alcohol? The first and most usual answer is **"NO!"** The subject of booze is a hard one. So many of our most pleasurable moments and memories are associated with it because of the society in which we live. A wedding without a toast to the bride and groom would not seem complete. The birth of a child is an occasion to be celebrated by raising a glass. An engagement, passing a driving test, winning a place at college. The list of times alcohol significantly enters our lives is endless, we could find an excuse to tipple every day. One of the favourite quotes of people who enjoy booze and seek an excuse, are the words of the apostle Paul in his letter to Timothy, "A little wine is good for the stomach." These words are true in the case of the average person, but not for someone with M.E. or Candida problems. Wine plays havoc with the intestinal flora. The yeast and sugar content will feed Candida faster than almost anything else because of this, wine is a very definite No! No!

Some people feel a meal with friends without a glass of wine is incomplete. They feel their friends will be slighted, offended by their refusal to imbibe. If they really are your friends, they will have your best interests and good health at heart, so they will understand when you explain the reason for your abstinence.

Beware of beer! Terrible! Made from yeast, sugar and malt, all things Candida flourishes on. Alcoholics frequently have serious Candida problems. This prompts one to ask, which came first, alcoholism or the Candida demanding to be fed.

Vodka and Gin are both distilled rather than fermented, having no sugar content, so on rare occasions, some sufferers may indulge in a tot because they do the least amount of damage. If you do, please be cautious. I have to add, it is better to abstain until you are well.

"Be brave, say no, stay well"

ALLERGIES - Living with them

Most of us at some time have been told by a physician who does not understand or know the answer to our problem, "You will just have to learn to live with it." Then he says "Next please."

Dismissed, confused and ill we wonder just how we are going to 'live with it.' People who have M.E., Candida and allergies are experiencing this dilemma. How does one live with a bewildering array of symptoms, the confusion of a weird diet, plus taking 20 different supplements daily? At the same time we may be reacting in a terrifying way to chemicals which our family and friends can tolerate. If this is a description of you, you will be used to being treated as a fanatic, hypochondriac or in need of a psychiatrist. What you really need is acceptance from others that your illness really does exist, more under-standing of it's symptoms and causes along with support while you do battle with it.

One of the things least understood, is the link between M.E., Candida and allergies. Allergy occurs when the immune system is weakened. M.E. and Candida are both immuno-deficiency diseases, therefore allergies are common to both. As the immune system is strengthened, allergies fade and eventually disappear. *So take heart, you can be normal again.*

Observation has led to the conclusion that not only antibiotics, birth control pills, and steroid treatments have led to these illnesses, but the entire spectrum of modern living. We have departed too far from natural things and substituted man-made items in all aspects of life.

Everything is derived from, or contaminated by, chemicals. Not just in the field of medicine and the food chain, but our entire environment has become alien to the needs of the human body. Let me explain...

Our bodies are constructed of atoms, little bundles of universal energy. By breathing and consuming more energy in the form of air, plant life and animals, we are able to sustain and replace energy as we burn it. Whilst these elements remain in their natural state, the human

23

body can assimilate these components and convert them into usable energy. When this is so, the energy flow between man and his environment remains balanced and all is well. If we interfere with the natural scheme of things, we rearrange the careful balance of energy levels needed to maintain good health.

Legislation is constantly being passed to safeguard the quality of our food. 'E' numbers on packaging helped, but not enough. The principle of genuine purity is being lost. Mankind has lost his way. B.S.E testifies to this. For as long as man has availed himself of cattle, they have chosen to roam free, and eat vegetation. Man interfered, feeding them with dead animal matter and immediately they became unfit for human consumption. Even on a totally organic diet, (if such a thing can now exist) allergies and sensitivities continue to multiply. Our bodies are being bombarded from all directions, air, water and the food chain are only some of the chemically contaminated elements making us ill.

Wisely reduce the overload as much as possible in your battle to restore healthy immune responses

How can it be done? Take a good look around your home, what do you see? Where once wood was used, now there is plastic, melamine or Formica. Where cotton, wool, hop-sack, silk, and linen used to be, nylon, polyester, Terylene and Dralon etc. have been substituted. Ask yourself, "What is the content of my carpet, curtains, three-piece-suite?" The answer in most cases will be, man made fibres. All giving off static electricity. In some homes and workplaces, people have experienced electric shocks from door handles, T.V. sets, computers, microwaves and many other items. You can, no doubt add to the list from your own experience. In some places it has become necessary to wear rubber soled shoes to insulate against serious shock.

How about your bed? Polyester sheets? Terylene duvet? Pillows, feather or man made? Foam filled mattress perhaps? What do you wear in bed? Nylon or polyester pyjamas? Even if only some of this is true you are subjecting your body to alien energy for at least eight hours a day whilst you sleep.

What about when you rise? Do you wear cotton underwear or easy care man-made fibres? How many items of your clothing are natural or are they all derived from chemicals? Do you have a body odour problem? If so, could it be your body protesting, "Get this off me"? Do you do your washing with biological detergents, or make the effort to use only soap powders? What do you use to clean the house? Chemicals in aerosol cans or natural soaps and waxes? Do you use antiperspirants, deodorants, hair sprays, perfumes and after shaves? Do you smoke? All these things are causing an unnatural imbalance of energy around your already overloaded body.

The way to speed up your recovery is to reduce the overload as much as possible. Don't become fanatical, there is no way to remove yourself from the planet entirely and you could risk alienating those around you who might otherwise be willing to help, but you can, slowly and sensibly change things, replacing with natural items. For instance, drink parsley tea instead of using a deodorant. Buy non-perfumed soap, change to a less exotic hairstyle that doesn't require spray. As you buy new clothes, select cotton, wool, silk and linen. You may not be able to afford so many, but your health will improve dramatically, and incidentally so will your temper, mine did.

I advise anyone experiencing severe chemical reactions to create a "haven" for themselves. A special room where everything is natural, where they can retreat from the world of irritants, and enjoy a short respite from the symptoms they cause.

The room should be stripped entirely and either emulsioned or papered (not vinyl). Floorboards need to be sealed with varnish and left bare. Several days must elapse before the room will be clear of decorating smells, but low odour products are becoming more readily available. Next you should furnish it with only natural items. Skin or wool rugs. Cotton curtains, shell, wicker, glass or paper lamp shades. Feather cushions with cotton covers, wooden furniture, polished only with beeswax. Add glass or wooden ornaments and your favourite books and your retreat is complete. No smoker or person wearing perfume may enter. You may choose to add a television or a music centre, but if you do, be sure to include a large piece of quartz crystal or the kind of plant that absorbs electromagnetic rays. (See Electromagnetism). One plant I am re-

25

ferring to is a cactus called Ceres Peruvianus, it eats the bad rays like the Venus fly trap eats flies. You may also find a dehumidifier and an ionizer will add to your comfort. Another indoor plant that is useful is the "Spider" plant. (Chlorophytum Comosum Var. Variegatum.)

These ideas don't have to cost a fortune, old furnishings are plentiful at auctions, second hand shops, jumble sales and car-boot sales. If you choose carefully, take them home and scrub them up, you will find great satisfaction in creating an attractive environment capable of paying you back with positive energy to help restore your depleted immune system.

"If you think this is all too much trouble, think how much trouble it is being ill, and how good it will be to recover and go back to a normal way of life, not being forced to 'live with it' any longer"

ALLERGY TESTS

There are a variety of tests available to determine the extent of your sensitivity to both food and chemicals, and it can be a veritable minefield to find your way through, culminating sometimes in a confused maze of things to avoid both coming in contact with and eating. *Many people miss the point of these tests. They look upon them as an end in themselves and assume that they must spend the rest of their lives avoiding the things identified as their personal allergens. This is a mistake.* The object of the exercise should be to identify the allergens to avoid for the time it takes to rebuild a strong immune system. Once the immune system is functioning well again, after appropriate treatment, another test will reveal whether it is safe to resume contact or consume the allergens originally identified, or not. This is a good measuring rod. It helps you determine how well your treatment is progressing. As time goes by, more and more of the original substances that caused you problems, should be revealed by the new tests, to have ceased to be problematic.

Some of the testing methods are:-
Applied Kinesiology
Blood tests
Hair analysis
Scratch tests
Vega machine

Of all these, I have found from experience that Applied Kinesiology is, (in the hands of a skilled practitioner) the most accurate, and my second choice would be Vega testing. This is based on similar testing of body energy, only through a machine. The other methods can turn out to be a bit 'hit and miss' so be careful which method you choose or *you could end up eating things you shouldn't, or being deprived of foods you need for good health.*

"A varied diet is vitamin rich"

ANTIBIOTICS

While you are unwell, you may contract an infection for which your doctor prescribes antibiotics. Ask yourself, are they really necessary?

Could there be an alternative way to treat the problem? (See the heading "Ways of avoiding drugs"). If you can find another way, try it first. You may be able to save yourself a lot of extra illness and money.

Let's take a closer look at the root meaning of the word antibiotic. First the Greek word 'anti' meaning to oppose, or against, and then 'bio' from the Greek word 'bios', meaning life, or living organisms. When you string the two meanings together you have the name given to a medication that is "against life," or in direct opposition to it.

Do you think you have enough life-force in you, at your low ebb, to risk destroying any more? If you already feel perpetually tired and listless, think what another course of antibiotics could do to you! Another point to consider is, if you are following the programme closely, you will be spending substantial amounts of money on a good probiotic (for life), (See the heading Probiotics), trying to re-establish the life force you lost. *A course of antibiotics could, in a few days, wipe out what it has taken you months to achieve.* However, antibiotics do have a place, but that place is at deaths door.

Weigh your situation carefully, and if you decide that a course of antibiotics are unavoidable, *then make sure you treble your intake of probiotic during the course and continue for a fortnight afterwards.* This will give you the best chance of maintaining the life balance you have gained up to that point. When Alexander Fleming discovered the use of penicillin (the first antibiotic), he recommended that live yoghurt be taken with it to counter balance its affect in the gut. Unfortunately this information has not been passed on to many patients. In any case, live yoghurt would not be sufficient to redress the problem in a patient who is already severely deficient. It has been estimated you would need at least eight pints (9.09 litres) a day to re-establish the balance. Your probiotic is cheaper and much less fattening.

"Avoid antibiotics and help your life force flourish"

AROMATHERAPY

Can aromatherapy clear a Candida problem or help with M.E.? Alone it can't, although used in conjunction with therapeutic massage it can bring great comfort, relieving aching muscles and joint pain. The oils, mixed carefully, by a knowledgeable masseur are invaluable for helping clear toxic waste during the 'die-off' stage of treatment. This is when the overgrowth of Candida is destroyed and begins to clog your system, causing a great deal of discomfort. (See Herxheimer Reaction.) A good lymphatic massage, skilfully performed, with the right mix of essential oils, will make the process easier to bear and speed up recovery if done on a regular basis. In the clinic I have found every two weeks is ideal, but monthly is still helpful if money is short.

A warning here to those experiencing this type of massage for the first time. If you are full of toxins, as most sufferers are at the outset, and your practitioner is doing the job correctly, you will feel 'off' for a few days afterwards. You may feel extremely tired and possibly think you have a virus. It is due to the rubbish in your system being on the move. Don't worry. Rest as much as possible and it will pass. When it does, you'll feel the benefits.

As well as massages, aromatherapy can be used internally. A variety of helpful preparations can be made to individual requirements to help alleviate unpleasant symptoms while the main programme is underway. This enables the sufferer to avoid the use of drugs and antibiotics. Do be sure your aromatherapist is skilled at mixing internal remedies as *essential oils are extremely strong and can be dangerous if not handled with caution.*

A blend of lavender, eucalyptus and camphor is recommended for the lymphatic massage mentioned above.

"Aromatherapy is an addition to, not a replacement for the supplement programme"

BACTERIA

When bacteria is mentioned we usually assume it is harmful, and much of it is. Bacteria are germs. Micro-organisms breed in billions. There are bad ones and good ones though, and the good ones are called by some 'friendly flora.' That's because they do invaluable work in the alimentary tract. When they are in proper balance in our gut they keep an inner harmony resulting in good health. If they become unbalanced then we become ill. The ones we are particularly concerned with for the purpose of this book are the pro-biotics, bifidus bifodum and Lactobaccillus acidophilus. I write much more extensively about them under the heading 'Probiotics.'

" 'Friendly flora' mean good health"

BELIEFS

Whatever your illness, your spirituality, or lack of it, can affect the kind of progress you make. Candida and M.E. are no exceptions.

In the Bible the apostle Paul made clear that emotions such as jealousy, anger and envies, coupled with enmity, contention and strife were not only ungodly, but self destructive.

He then listed, love, joy, peace, long-suffering, kindness, goodness, self control, mildness and faith as being beneficial. (See Galatians 5 v 19 to 21).

Solomon, credited with great wisdom said, "A calm heart is life to the flesh." (see Proverbs 14 v 30).

Both of them were, and still are right. Each time you allow yourself to succumb to destructive emotions, your heart rate and blood pressure rise, adrenaline is released and this in turn causes your blood sugar level to increase, feeding your Candida problem from within.

So what you believe, and how you live your beliefs, has a great bearing on your health. If you strive to live peaceably, you will alleviate the aggression of others around you, therefore reducing stresses and tensions so commonplace in the world we live in. Not only will you benefit others, but you will gain yourself, and good health will be your reward.

"Be calm, be peaceable, be loving and be well"

BOWEL - see Colon

CANDIDA - What is it?

Candida albicans is what its Latin name implies, a white fungus. It is a parasite present in the human gut from birth onward. Under normal conditions it is kept under control by "friendly flora" or useful bacteria who make their home in the human alimentary tract. These friendly bacteria or Probiotics as they have become known, are essential for good health. They keep the natural balance of things right and ensure our immune system stays healthy. One very powerful strain is bifidus bifodum. This is the first friendly bacterium to enter our system by means of mothers milk. It lines the gut and under natural conditions will ensure a healthy immune system for life. Between the ages of five and seven it is joined by L.acidophilus, completing the weaning process and equipping the human immune system to cope with increasing demands made by adult life on immune responses. Of course these are not the only friendly bacteria in our bodies, there are many others, but these are the ones primarily involved in ensuring good health by helping to control parasites, particularly Candida albicans. If these bacteria are destroyed, then the Candida fungi is permitted to multiply unrestrained. When this happens, the fungi buds and forms clusters, eventually attaching itself to the walls of the intestines. It then begins to grow fine, hair like structures, penetrating the gut wall and causing perforations. (See illustrations 1 and 2 on page 35)

The second stage is called the mycelial stage. This is when serious problems can begin. The gut can now leak its contents into the blood stream. When leakage is from the colon, the most common site of the problem, poisons destined to be expelled from the body, now seep though to contaminate the bloodstream, carrying with them microscopic spores capable of traveling and multiplying throughout the body. In fact everywhere blood travels the Candida spores will try to establish a new site in which to thrive. This has become known as 'Leaky Gut Syndrome.' It is the time when the sufferer begins to feel extremely fatigued and generally ill all over. It explains why the symptoms arising from candidiasis are so many and varied. Very few people realize the strong connection between this stage of candida overgrowth and ulcerative colitis, inflammatory bowel disease and irritable bowel syndrome.

It also explains why the immune system comes under attack, gradually ceasing to protect the sufferer from alien substances. This is the link between Candida albicans and allergy. As immunity diminishes allergies develop.

The uncontrolled parasite can move freely through the alimentary tract, causing all sorts of intestinal and digestive problems. Among them may be counted heartburn, indigestion, malabsorption, hiatus hernia, thrush, both oral and vaginal, adhesions in the intestines, causing pains resembling appendicitis, constipation and worm infestation, also making way for other destructive parasites. It can travel from the rectum to the vagina, enter the womb and contribute to endometriosis and a variety of menstrual problems. From the vagina along to the urethra, up into the kidney to cause cystitis and other kidney infections. Wherever it travels it leaves havoc and misery in it's wake. Men can infect their sex partners if they carry it under the foreskin, or have a fungal infection around the groin. (Called by Americans 'jock itch'). Women can likewise infect their partners. It just gets tossed back and forth between the two unless both are treated simultaneously.

Yes Candida can, and does, cause myriad symptoms, some trivial, but others extremely serious. If left undetected and untreated it can lead to life threatening circumstances. Cancer research has established a definite connection and every A.I.Ds patient has a serious overgrowth. Check the symptom list in this book.

If you think you have an overgrowth, do something now.

"Control Candida and avoid ailments"

A simple illustration of Candida overgrowth in the colon

Figure 1

A healthy colon with normal Candida albicans fungi (depicted as egg shapes) surrounded and controlled by 'friendly flora' (depicted as dots).

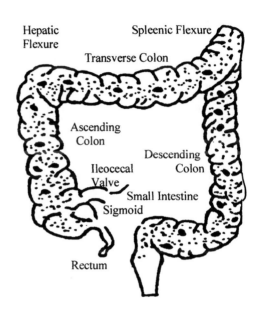

Hepatic Flexure

Spleenic Flexure

Transverse Colon

Ascending Colon

Descending Colon

Ileocecal Valve

Small Intestine

Sigmoid

Rectum

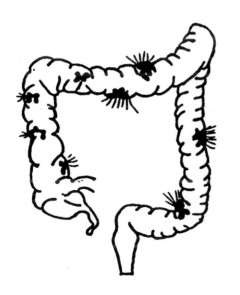

Figure 2

What happens when the fungi is unrestrained and reaches the mycelial form.

A) The yeast like phase when it reproduces by budding.

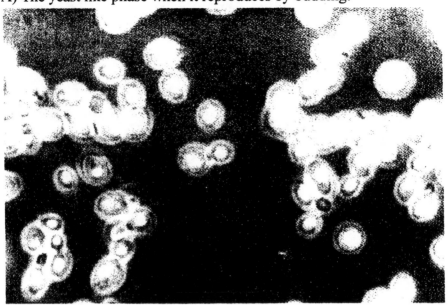

These are photographs taken of Candida under a microscope by Dr. Micheal Tuite, Senior lecturer in Molecular Biology at the University of Kent, Canterbury. England.

B) As it changes from the yeast to the mycelial phase.

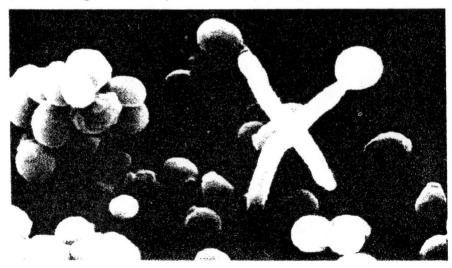

CAUSES OF CANDIDIASIS

The massive and repeated doses of antibiotics administered indiscriminately for a multitude of minor ailments over the last few decades, has of course made a major contribution to the epidemic. (At the time of writing, estimates indicate one in three people world wide have an overgrowth to some extent.) At the same time, women are urged to take birth control pills, implants and the morning after pill, all of which result in depleted zinc and magnesium levels in their bodies. This in turn leads eventually to immune breakdown. Children born after extended use of these birth control methods are born deficient in these two, and other essential trace elements. Some young women find it impossible to conceive, whilst those who do, cannot pass on to their offspring an inheritance they themselves do not possess.

Breast milk from an ex-birth pill, implant user or someone repeatedly treated with antibiotics may also be deficient in valuable bifidus bifodum so essential for the formation and establishment of a healthy immune system in the infant. The lack of this bacterium is particularly manifest in those born between 1920 and the early 1960's because, in the so called civilized world, it was unfashionable to breast feed. Thankfully the trend has changed, but these other factors are rendering breast milk impotent anyway. Hormone replacement therapy, other hormone treatments and steroids are having similar effects. Is it any wonder more allergies are developing in our day than at any other time in human history?

Add to this the use of hormones, steroids and antibiotics in raising animals for human consumption, and you may begin to see the extent of the problem. Factory farming with its use of chemical fertilizers and sprays is another contributory factor. Smoking, not only makes the smoker more susceptible to fungal overgrowth, but also weakens others sharing the same air space. Airborne fumes of all kinds are affecting our immune systems. Radiation must take a share of the blame, as must electromagnetism from computers, television sets, mobile telephones, microwave ovens and power cables etc... Take into the equation the destruction of the ozone layer and a host of other man made "miracles" and the problem becomes increasingly more apparent.

A major new factor in the causes of Candida overgrowth is the destruction of the ozone layer. Rainfall and humidity levels have escalated allowing perfect conditions for mould overgrowth as flood waters recede. (See heading, Climate-does it effect you?)

If man is to survive his technological advances, he must learn to protect himself from the devastating affects. For ways of combating these problems. (See the heading, Allergies - Living with them).

The programme recommended in this book is designed to bring your Candida level back to normal so you can be well again, but there is no absolute guarantee it will stay under control for the rest of your life, because of the world we live in. However, once you have learned the rules, you will recognize a return of symptoms early on and take steps to prevent yourself from becoming seriously ill again.

None of us will remain well unless the causes of the epidemic are removed.

They are:-
Chemical and Technological Pollution Worldwide.

"Control the causes and reap the reward of good health"

CLIMATE - does it effect you?

Many people report they feel terrible on a damp, rainy day, but are really improved when the sun shines. They ask me if there is a reason for this. Thinking of the nature of the illness, and applying logic leads to the conclusion that there is. Fungi likes and flourishes in damp places. On the shady side of a tree, under the sink, the bottom of the shower curtain, in fact anywhere there are warm, damp conditions it grows prolifically. On the other hand you will rarely, if ever, see fungus when the sun is shining and dry conditions prevail. Candida is a fungi, therefore it behaves like all the others. Do try to avoid damp, musty places. They really will make you feel very ill.

Climatic changes caused by the destruction of the ozone layer have led to the "greenhouse effect." This has meant global warming causing increased rainfall and humidity. In many places flood waters have encroached on peoples living space leaving dampness and mould growth. The spores released into the air can be very harmful to health for everyone, but particularly to those who have Candida overgrowth already. If necessary, be prepared to abandon contaminated possessions in order to preserve good health, and move to higher ground if possible.

Many of my clients, after taking holidays in warm dry climates, return feeling much better. Hence my recommendation is to seek the sun whenever possible, even if you only manage a few minutes a day in a sunny room. It really will help.

"Keep your sunny side up"

COLON

The colon is the name given to the large intestine running from the ileum to the anus. In the diagram on the following page the colon is marked heavily in black. In Eastern medicine it is considered **THE** most important part of the body since on its function, the health and well being of the entire body depends. It is the waste disposal unit. Everything we eat is broken down into a fluid called chyme during the digestive process. The goodness utilizable by the body is extracted as it passes through the alimentary tract. Finally, what is left is disposable waste. The ileo cecal valve now opens to allow the fluid to pass from the small intestine into the colon, where it will form faeces in the bowel, ready to be expelled from the body.

It is in the colon that Candida originates and it is there, it gets out of control.

When the balance of colonic bacteria is lost, the troubles start. Candida overgrowth can be the direct cause of antonia of the bowel, irritable bowel syndrome, colitis, diverticulitis, Crohns disease and many other serious conditions. When bowel function is impaired, toxic waste can seep into the blood stream resulting in poisoning of the entire body.

A clean colon and a *regular bowel movement* is an *absolute must for a healthy body.* By 'regular bowel movement' I mean, *at least once a day.* It has become commonplace for physicians to tell their patients, if they go once or twice a week, it is all right if it is normal for you. I disagree adamantly! If you eat good food with a proper content of roughage three times a day, you should defecate almost as often. If you don't, something is very wrong. Look at your dietary intake. Add more fibre and bulk by consuming more whole foods such as brown rice, bran, skins and green, leafy, fresh vegetables. If you are allowed fruit, add more prunes or figs. If that doesn't work, take a gentle herbal laxative until clearance is achieved and proper daily function is restored. There are colon cleansing products available to help, specially formulated to include 'friendly' bacteria along with fibrous bulk and cleansing herbs. Since bifido bifodum is the predominant friendly microorganism inhabiting the large intestine, (makes up 85% of the stool bulk and absorbs and transports the waste), the oral and anal use of this bacterium has amazing results on both constipation and diarrhoea. There is also a product containing butyric acid to help heal perforations in the colon.

So, if you'll pardon the expression,

"Get moving"

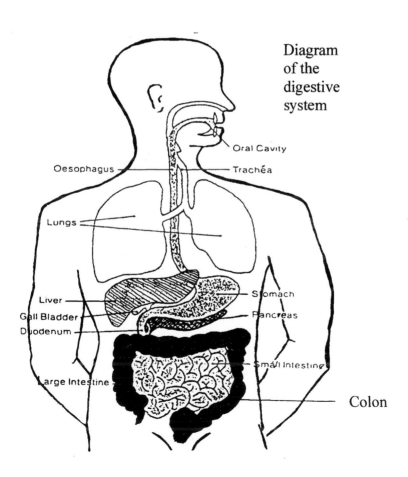

Diagram
of the
digestive
system

Oral Cavity

Oesophagus — *Trachéa*

Lungs

Liver

Gall Bladder

Duodenum

Stomach

Pancreas

Small Intestine

Large Intestine

Colon

COLONIC IRRIGATION

Much credence has been given to this practice and I am sure it has had its successes, but I do think it should be approached with great caution. To pump litres of water into the body from the wrong end seems, to say the least, a little unnatural. The theory is, this will clear the colon of impacted faeces and impurities and thereby restore cleanliness and proper bowel function, thus improving the clients health and general vitality. Among the impurities cleansed from the colon would, it is claimed, be Candida albicans overgrowth. This maybe so, but unless a regime of dietary restrictions and supportive supplements is followed, there will be an immediate recurrence of the problem. Also, if the Candida and impurities are washed away, so too is the "friendly flora." *Re-population of the colon must be done after each treatment.*

A point to consider is, having a pipe inserted into the rectum by a virtual stranger may prove distasteful and distressing to some people. I think that particular stress should be avoided if possible.

Another danger is, if the condition has already reached the mycelial stage, the water will force the Candida spores through the perforations in the colon wall, causing the problem to travel further throughout the system. The client may then end up in a worse condition than when they started. I have seen this happen many times.

There may, however, be a time when colonic irrigation will be helpful, but in my view, it should be a very last resort and then it must only be administered by an extremely competent practitioner.

If more help than a gentle laxative is needed, my recommendation is to use a self administered enema. An enema kit can be obtained from Earthdust products. (See Useful Addresses).

"It will be all right in the end"

COMMUNICATION

One of the most common phrases uttered by Candida and M.E. sufferers is "Nobody understands how I feel." Of course they don't. How can they unless they too have the same illness? It is possible though, to help others be more sympathetic, if you learn to communicate your problems adequately. Often we expect others to understand immediately a subject of which they have no knowledge at all. If you look back you will realize, it took you yourself quite a long time to understand your problem, and you were living with it daily. So don't expect too much of others too soon. What you need to do is, think out and plan carefully how best to explain about the condition as simply, briefly and pleasantly as possible. You want to enlist the aid of those around you, not alienate them.

Do try not to perpetually moan and groan about your symptoms. You already appear to them to be 'faddy' about your food. Try not to bend their ear about the finer points of allergic reactions to foods, let it suffice to say something like, "Thank you, but I must refuse because it makes me ill. I know you wouldn't want that." This makes them think carefully about what is being offered. They may even have visions of you throwing up on their carpet, but you won't go on and on and bore them to death with the lurid details. Of course, if they ask more about it, you will then know that they are truly interested, and what you say won't irritate them. Watch carefully for the first signs of them losing interest and then stop.

After all, you don't need the understanding of everybody on earth. It should be enough to have the sympathy of your nearest and dearest, and to know your practitioner is on your wavelength.

You may find this book useful to explain your health problems to others, but if you would like something shorter, I have produced a more concise, 40 page booklet, helpful to give or to loan to busy people like doctors, employers, health visitors etc... If you would like a copy, contact the publisher at the address in the front of this book (page 1) and one will be sent to you. At the time of going to press, the price is £2.50 including pp.

So when you want understanding, try communicating by asking people questions about themselves. Everybody likes to expound on the subject of "me." They will think you such a pleasant person, they will be glad to listen to you the next time you need understanding about your health problem.

If you feel you really must talk extensively to someone about your problems, why not join a support group? There are quite a few springing up now, but do be sure you don't end up becoming thoroughly depressed by continually bringing health problems to the fore in your mind, or by being 'agony aunt' to all the other members of the group. *Remember, uplifting subjects will crowd out the miseries.*

"The only way to have a friend is to be one"

"Who hears me, who understands me, becomes mine"
Ralph Waldo Emerson

CRAVING - for goodies

"I am desperate for a chocolate bar," or "I'd murder for a slice of bread and marmite." These are common cries in the early stages of the Candida, M.E. programme. The reason for this terrible urge to eat what is forbidden on your diet is because you have begun depriving the Candida of the very things it needs in order to multiply and survive. Chocolate, milk and sugar. Bread and marmite both contain yeast.

When you stop eating these things you not only hit the fungi hard with the diet, but at the same time your anti-fungal supplement is killing it off too. No wonder it sets up a craving for the foods it depends on for survival. The parasite is fighting for it's life. *Don't let it win by giving in.* If you do, you will have undone all the good you have achieved up to that point and will have to start all over again. If you manage to sit it out, you will find the cravings lessen and eventually stop in a few days.

Some people, when they come to the end of the treatment period, try to take sugary, milky, yeasty foods again. They find they taste like poison, which is exactly what "goodies" have become to them.

Never allow cravings to get out of hand again and you will control Candida for the rest of your life.

"Fight back and feel fine soon"

CYSTITIS

This condition plagues so many people suffering from Candida and M.E. It has been described as sheer misery to me, in the clinic. One lady said she felt as though she was "peeing broken glass." It must be awful. What can you do about it in the short term? We have found loose panties of cotton or silk, not man-made fibre helps. Tights should be avoided. Wear stockings and a suspender belt or crutchless tights if you can find some. Sunday papers often advertise these garments for other purposes.

When you feel an attack starting, *drink several litres of water.* Yes, that's what I said, litres. *At least four litres a day.* This will flush the kidneys through and hopefully wash out the infection. Water can be taken as barley water or parsley tea, both have been found helpful by herbalists for their beneficial effects on the kidneys. Plain bottled or filtered water is good too, but avoid tap water if at all possible.

As cystitis is one of the predominant symptoms of Candida infection, attacks should become less as treatment progresses. Some sufferers have found attacks cease immediately they stop having any form of sugar, but return when they begin eating fruit again after the first month on the regime. If this happens to you, keep off fruit for as long as it takes to clear your kidneys of the problem. Only resume eating it cautiously after a longer period of treatment with the supplements.

One fruit found to be allowable and helpful is cranberry. It has been found to have helpful properties in prevention of 'E' coli, the bacteria partially responsible for infection leading to an attack of cystitis, from adhering to the bladder wall.

Cranberry is also available as a very helpful product combined with L. acidophilus powder.

"Water helps to wash it away"

DAILY ROUTINE

It is hard to stress enough the importance of making and keeping to a set routine.

It is an important part of your battle back to health.

While you are feeling your worst, you will find 'routine' difficult because it is then, that everything seems impossible, but whatever happens, don't stop trying. Have a set time to do things and stick to it. If you don't, the day will slide by and your memory will have robbed you of something necessary to your regime.

1st:- Make a list   2nd:- Follow it

The very first thing on your agenda must be to take your bacterium. When you wake, your stomach is empty. This is the time you will gain most benefit from it. Why not pop the jar, straight from the fridge, into a wide necked thermos flask and take it to bed with you, together with a glass of spring water. When you wake, you can mix it and settle back in your pillows, taking your time to come to.

It is a fact, if you can struggle out of bed, wash, shave (if male), do your hair and dress neatly, you will feel more able to face the day. So do it next. Your bacterium will be working away whilst you are.

Now have your breakfast and the rest of the supplements. Whilst you have all the packs out, count out the other doses to see you through the day, wrapping them separately in foil, cling film or pop them into individual pill boxes. Place them into your bag or pocket, then wherever you are when the next dose is due, you will have them at hand.

You are now ready to battle your way through the day.

Lunch will be your next hurdle. If you go to work you will need to have thought ahead about what is obtainable for a meal nearby. If there is nowhere close to provide something suitable, you will have to prepare something to take with you. Either last thing at night, or directly after breakfast.

With a little forethought it is possible to have quite a variety of nourishing cold meals. Why not have a look at the recipe section in this publication or obtain a copy of my book "Cooking for Candida," where there are fantastic ideas for packed lunches. The emphasis must be on quick preparation, easy availability and light to carry.

Don't forget to take your midday supplements.

Eat your evening meal as early as possible to allow your stomach to be empty for your second dose of bacterium before bedtime.

Make evening times as restful as possible. Let friends visit you, or you them. It will lift your spirits, but don't make the visits too long. People with the best intentions in the world can sap your energy. You need all the energy you have to get well. Don't spend your evenings in smoky atmospheres. If members of your household smoke, ask them kindly to refrain from doing so in the same room as you. Or discreetly retreat to another room. Go to bed at a reasonable hour. Even if you have difficulty sleeping, your body will benefit from being rested. Rest as much as you can.

Whatever happens, *plan your day, make it fit your needs.* Juggle with it until it is working well for you, not against you. Then *stick to your schedule.* You will benefit in so many ways.

"Routine is rewarding"

DENTAL TREATMENT

A visit to the dentist can be a traumatic experience for anyone, but it becomes more so when you are ill. Especially for those who are trying to avoid chemicals and antibiotics. My advice is, stay away as long as you dare, to give your immune system as long as possible to recover and be strengthened by the treatment programme. When you eventually do go, you will be less likely to suffer bad reactions to the anaesthetic injections used. If however, it simply can't be avoided, then *Make a point of telling your dentist about your problem.* He is much more familiar with candidiasis than the average doctor. He will have seen it often in the form of oral thrush. Also he will be aware of just how difficult it is to treat.

There are now a better range of products available for the dentist to choose from in order to treat you alternatively. Not only are there non mercury substitutes for amalgam fillings, but also special anaethetics for use on those experiencing allergic reactions. Discuss the use of one of these before your treatment begins. He may then choose from Prilocaine, Mepivacaine, Citanest, or Articaine. Articaine is proving the most successful in avoiding adrenaline related reactions.

Much publicity has been given to the problem of amalgam fillings releasing mercury into the system, slowly causing poisoning and possible mental problems. Some Candida and M.E. sufferers have had dramatic improvement of many of their symptoms by having amalgams removed and replaced with composite fillings, or composite and porcelain inlay. If you choose this approach to your problem, be very careful who you select to carry out the dental work. If the procedure is not carried out in a specific way, then worsening of symptoms can result. If you are making good progress toward good health, then mercury is not a problem and you may be best advised to leave well alone. Only if you fail to improve after following the regime for four months, should you give consideration to the possibility that your amalgam fillings could be the reason you are making little headway. Vega or kinesiology tests can, in the hands of an experienced practitioner, identify the mercury leakage for you. Tests can also be carried out to find which teeth need treating, if any, thus saving you money on unnecessary dental work.

If you give the matter proper thought you will take into account that mercury is one of the most toxic substances known to man, second only to plutonium, so why has it been used extensively as a large part (about 52%) of the amalgam mix used for dental fillings. Does it not seem odd to place a poisonous substance into the mouth only inches from the brain.

Dentist have protested since the 1800s that when mercury is mixed with copper, tin silver and zinc to make up the silver fillings we have all become accustomed to, it does not escape and therefore is not a threat to health. Evidence is mounting to the contrary. A tie up is being established between such diseases as Alzheimer's, M.S. Candidiasis, multiple allergy syndrome and M.E. Mercury has even been found to accumulate in the foetus of the unborn child when pregnant women have dental treatment during pregnancy.

It could be that many obscure health problems, formerly gone undiagnosed could be connected with seepage of mercury from old amalgam fillings.

If you do decide to go ahead and have yours removed, you should be aware that there are precautions to be observed, or you could make yourself even worse than you already are. There are now mercury free dental practices springing up everywhere. For lists of those who are aware of the right procedure, you can contact Dr. Jack Levenson, President of the British Dental Society for Clinical Nutrition. He has also written a very comprehensive book on the subject called "Menace in the Mouth."

Also in the U.S.A., Hal Huggins book on the subject 'It's All in Your Head' is well worth reading before making decisions. (See Useful Addresses)

"Take care of your teeth
and they will take care of you"

DESENSITIZATION

This form of treatment should be given great thought. Administered by a competent practitioner, it can greatly reduce the severity of allergic reactions, which will be of great value if the reactions are of life threatening proportions. However it does nothing to correct the initial causes of the sensitivities.

For instance, the sufferer may have been eating repetitively and taking vast amounts of unwise foods throughout their lives. Unless he or she is prepared to rethink their eating habits, the problem will keep recurring.

Neither will desensitization make up deficiencies in the body. These may have been the major cause of the breakdown in the immune system initially.

If repeated antibiotic, hormone and steroid treatments have been administered over a long period of time, the only way to redress the balance will be a long course of probiotic and vitamin treatment to feed and strengthen the immune system. It is far wiser to correct the causes, than to screen off reactions designed to warn you that all is not well.

When this is done, you will be able to have contact with your particular allergen without having a bad reaction.

It can take up to three years for the immune system to recover it's resilience, not only to food and drugs, but also to environmental chemicals and pollutants. Don't bombard your body with substances it is trying to tell you to avoid.

"Keep away from your allergens and feed the deficiencies.
Eventually you will regain a healthy immune response"

DIAGNOSIS

Before embarking on any form of treatment, be sure you really do have Candida or M.E. Many of the symptoms are similar to each other but can also be associated with a number of other diseases. It would be easy to self diagnose and assume your symptoms are due to Candida albicans or M.E. when you could be suffering from something else entirely. Let your doctor test for other problems in order to eliminate them. Only when everything has proved negative should you take on the M.E. or Candida label. It would be terrible if you neglected to seek treatment for a life threatening condition until it was too late.

When everything else has finally been ruled out, and you are tired of being told you are imagining it all, then is the time to seek out a competent complementary practitioner for a definite diagnosis.

Some doctors are now recognizing M.E. quite readily but few will acknowledge systemic candidiasis and therefore often confuse the two. Don't argue, because the vitamins, minerals and bacteria needed are the same in both cases. In some places the state medical system can prescribe them, but don't expect too much.

There are many different methods of diagnosis, blood tests, iridology, reflexology, saliva tests, applied kinesiology, food allergy patterns, Vega tests, Mora tests etc... In fact the methods of diagnosis are almost as many as the symptoms. The true test of a positive diagnosis is, if the treatment works. Then you know the diagnosis was correct. It all depends on finding a practitioner who's experience and judgment you can trust.

"When you know what it is. Decide what to do about it, then do it"

DIE OFF - see Herxheimer

DIET

Eating is one of the major delights of living, not just a necessity of life. It ranks with log fires, hot baths and the joys of love making. Along with those others, it deserves to be given time and a degree of reverence. Food is a gift from God. To be deprived of it is a terrible hardship, therefore I understand when people say, "Oh! Please don't put me on a diet." Or, "I can't eat that, I've never liked it." I understand, but I don't let them get away with it.

When your health is at stake, you *must* review your attitude to food. I'm including a few basic principles. Principles are different from rules, they allow room for variation and individuality, leaving you free to experiment with your own ideas, within those principles. In this way you will be encouraged to develop eating habits to last a lifetime, ensuring you regain your health but also enabling you to enjoy every meal you prepare. Remember, it isn't just what you cook but the way you present it that makes a meal appetizing.

There are a million and more tastes you have yet to experience. If one food must be rejected for health reasons, there will be many alternatives to choose from to take it's place. Be adventurous. Try new foods. If you become allergic to strawberries, try a mango, or kiwi next time you visit the supermarket. If onions are ruled out, reach for a leek. Titillate your taste buds with foods from foreign lands. Soon you will be enjoying a whole new eating experience, and at the same time you will be regaining your health. Each food carries a variety of vitamins and minerals to help you.

I shall only state briefly the things you mustn't have. They are important, but don't let us be negative. What you *can* eat is the important thing.

Often when told about the diet, people complain "But there is nothing left to eat." Pure nonsense! The earth produces an abundance of food in a profusion of varieties. It is because people become accustomed to repetitive eating, they forget how to choose, and so don't know how to prepare what they consider as 'strange foods'. I am astonished by the number of people who come into my kitchen and, when seeing pulses in jars exclaim, "I wouldn't know what to do with those." The answer is, find out. If you can read, you can educate yourself on any subject under the sun.

A healthy diet is your passport to future well being so don't discard the whole programme because of the *restriction of only three items.* There are substitutes for all three and I shall suggest a simple to follow, seven day diet plan to start you off, a few pages further on in this book. It won't be long before you start concocting mouthwatering goodies to replace your boring old diet, the diet that was making you ill, remember....

The Three Golden Rules.

1) No yeast, or foods based on fermentation.
2) No sugars of any kind, including honey.
3) No cows milk.

These are the essential things to avoid, but as an individual you may have become aware of allergic reactions or sensitivities to other foods. If so, you must adapt the following diet to your own particular needs. For example, if you react badly to onions, when the recipe calls for onions, leave them out and substitute leeks or garlic. It is extremely unlikely you will be allergic to all three. Perhaps your problem is wheat allergy. Replace wheat with buckwheat, bulgar wheat, potato, soya corn, rye, oats etc. There are many different flours to try. It may be you are not reacting to the wheat itself, but to the chemicals used in growing it, so a change to organic flour may solve your problem.

Since it is important to avoid chemicals, use as much organically grown food as possible. I realize this may be difficult, or even an impossibility in your locality. Don't think you have automatically failed, just do your best. All the changes you make will help to bring improvement. If you think you have a food allergy, but can't identify it, then Vega testing or Applied Kinesiology will identify it for you.

Now let's take these food bans one at a time and reason why they must be omitted from your diet.

Yeast... Since Candida is itself a yeast, and you already have an overgrowth, it makes sense to stop adding to the problem by eliminating all yeast from your menu. Your object is to reduce the yeast in your system.

Sugars... Sugar feeds yeast as any baker or wine maker knows. Have you ever watched bread rise, or wine ferment? If you have, then you will be aware of how quickly fermentation takes place. Bread can double in size in a matter of minutes when set to 'prove'. The same happens when Candida is fed with sugar. Is it any wonder you feel bloated. Your abdomen swells up just like a loaf. Not only that, but sugar helps create poisons which lead on to a variety of aches and pains. Avoid it like plague.

Cows milk ... Cows milk is very high in lactose, which is another form of sugar, therefore it feeds your Candida problem in the same way as other sugars, but there is much more to consider. Factory farming has led to cattle being fed unnaturally. A cow's natural food is grass, yet in recent years cattle have been fed on all manner of other things, including other dead animals. B.S.E. has been the result. You must question whether milk is still a food fit for human consumption. It is also common for cattle to be given hormones and antibiotics to improve milk yield and growth rate and fight infection. Milk is not what it used to be. Women perhaps, understand this better than men if they are mothers who have experience of breast feeding. They know whatever they eat or take into their bodies affects the quality of the breast milk. For instance, if a nursing mum eats too many plums, her baby may develop diarrhoea.

Steer clear of cow's milk and all dairy products made from it, like cheese, butter, cream, yoghurt etc. This doesn't mean no dairy products at all. You can have goat and sheep milk cheeses and yoghurt providing you have no personal sensitivity to them. Do be careful when buying Greek sheep yoghurt, some makes have cow's cream added so read the labels carefully. Also watch out for added whey powder in all sorts of products. This is milk too. It is sad to think God gave His people, "A land flowing with milk and honey" to ensure their health and prosperity, and man has contaminated this earth to the extent that those two valuable foods have become like poison to so many people.

These are some of the reasons why you should avoid these three basic foods. It will also be helpful to include a list of other named contents to keep clear of, because they will also cause the Candida yeast to multiply.

The following items can also stimulate Candida over-growth, so be sure to avoid them. Artificial sweeteners, glucose, syrups, dextrose, fructose. Malt, vinegars, avoid fruit and fruit juices but only only for the first month. Dried fruit should be bought with great caution as it often contains mould. The same is true of nuts which are not fresh. Buy them both wrapped in cellophane rather than polythene. Polythene encourages rotting and therefore fungi is produced along with fermentation. Avoid fungi forming foods such as mushrooms, peanuts, yeast based foods like breads and bun's, even some commercially produced pitta bread may include yeast. Yeast spreads such as marmite, vecon, bovril, alcohol, soya sauce and miso. Monosodium glutamate, gravy mixes and stock cubes with yeast, added preservatives, all artificial colourants, sweeteners and flavourings. Grapes because the bloom on them is a natural yeast. Hydrogenated vegetable oils.

When you change your eating habits, you may experience withdrawal symptoms such as, headaches, tummy discomfort, cravings for yeasty, sweet foods and possibly a general feeling of lassitude. More usually though great improvement is gained. Often people assume it will continue, but it only lasts until the die-off begins (See Herxheimer Reaction). The temptation is to blame the diet for making you feel unwell, as an excuse to break it.

Don't do it. Just keep going and it won't be long before you achieve genuine, lasting improvement.

SUGGESTED SEVEN DAY DIET PLAN

Sunday

Breakfast

Home made Muesli:- Oats, sunflower seeds, pumpkin seeds, flaked almonds, (toss all ingredients together in a container and shake) with soya, goat or sheep milk.

Lunch

Omelette with onions, garlic, mixed salad and baked potato.

Dinner

Roast lamb with garlic slotted into the flesh, greens (brassicas), carrots, and roast potatoes. Gravy made from yeast free stock cubes, add lamb juices, and thicken with corn flour.

Vegetarian alternative

Stir-fry with olive oil. Include bean shoots, courgettes, white or red cabbage, onions, garlic, sweet corn, carrots, peppers, tinned water chestnuts, and precooked rice. Add a sprinkling of curry powder to taste.

Monday

Breakfast

Scrambled eggs made with non-dairy margarine and soya, goat or sheep milk, on Ryvita, rice cakes or oat cakes (for wheat allergic use only Original Ryvita).

Lunch

Home made soup:- 1 celery stick, 1 onion, 1 carrot, garlic, mixed herbs, 425ml (¾pint) water, yeast free stock cube or powder. Cook all together for 20 minutes. Thicken with corn flour. Eat as it is with crackers or soda-bread, or purée.

Dinner

Yesterdays leftover cold lamb with either salad and cold new potatoes or fresh vegetables and mashed potatoes.

Vegetarian alternative

Vegetable Lasagne with baked potato.

Tuesday

Breakfast   Oatmeal porridge (made with water sheep, goat or soya milk), add soya or oat bran. Fruit after first month.

Lunch   Jacket potato with vegetable margarine and veg. cheese, (if no sensitivity), and side-salad. Or sheep/goat cheese.

Dinner   Free range chicken breast as Chicken Kiev using vegetable margarine and garlic as filling with a varied salad. Coat with oatmeal to avoid bread crumbs, and deep-fry in olive oil.

Vegetarian alternative   Bean casserole with home made pitta-bread.

Wednesday

Breakfast   Puffed rice (sugar free) with goat, sheep or soya milk (fruit after the first month).

Lunch   Tinned pilchards or mackerel in brine (check no additives) and mixed salad.

Dinner   Lambs liver with onions, garlic, greens, carrots and potatoes.

Vegetarian alternative   Home made pizza on a pastry base with vegetarian, sheep or goat cheese and mixed salad.

Thursday

Breakfast   Home made muesli and soya milk (see Monday). Fruit after the first month.

Lunch

Country soup mix (dried mixed pulses and barley. Available in most supermarkets) mix with 425ml (¾pint) of water and add yeast free stock cube. Eat with yeast free bread substitute (pitta, scofa or soda bread).

Dinner	Grilled fish with a knob of dairy free margarine and crushed garlic, chips done in olive oil and frozen broad beans.
Vegetarian alternative	Brown rice risotto with an abundance of feta cheese diced and added last.

Friday

Breakfast	Goat or sheep milk yoghurt. After first month add fruit.
Lunch	Rice cakes with hummus, raw carrot, celery sticks with onion rings. Dip them in hummus.
Dinner	Casseroled chicken breast with parsnip, turnip, swede, onion, garlic, any other vegetable desired. ½ lt (1pint) of filtered water and yeast free stock cube. Add dumplings of self raising flour and vegetable suet during last 20 minutes of cooking time.
Vegetarian alternative	Same as above minus chicken and adding pulses.

Saturday

Breakfast	Puffed rice (sugar free) with soya goat or sheep milk (fruit may be added after first month).
Lunch	Baked potato in jacket with salad.
Dinner	Trout, steak or chicken with variety of vegetables or salad and baked, boiled or chipped potatoes (today is purposely vague in case you go out for a meal, even fish and chips would be O.K). If you are at home, tuna fish in supreme sauce would be nice and easy.
Vegetarian alternative	Pasta and Italian tomato and garlic sauce with onion. Add other vegetables of your choice, or bean-burgers (see recipe section), and salad. If you are out, an omelette may be available.

Drinks:- Vegetable juices, spring water, (preferably bottled in glass) filtered water, carbonated spring water. Reputable herbal teas, Earl Grey, barley cup, dandelion coffee, Aqua Libra, Piermont, Perrier water, Sorelle, Tah-he-bo or Pau D'Arco tea, hot yeast free vegetable broth. Spring water with added fruit juice after the first month. Boiled water is not good, as boiling does not remove the chlorine (see the heading Water).

You will notice I have omitted wheat from the diet. I have done this because it is, along with milk, one of the most common allergens, and I thought it would help some of those who suffer from reactions to it, not to have to think out a special plan for themselves. Add wheat if you are O.K. on it. The diet is ***not a slimming diet*** so eat as much as you like of the foods you are allowed. You will probably lose weight anyway if you are overweight when you start, and if you are under weight you will possibly gain some; it can work both ways. The way it is planned is to ensure a good balance of nutrition, at the same time not being too repetitive. You can of course juggle it about to suit your personal needs, and as you get used to living without the yeast, milk and sugar, you will probably think of other combinations of food to add to it. You will find a variety of suitable ideas for different meal times in the 'Recipe' section of this book and even more in the publication "Cooking for Candida" by Jo Hampton. (Available from Kingston House Publishing, ISBN 0-9521544-1-2. See page one for address).

While I approve of vegetarianism, I find it unwise to insist on it when your diet is restricted, unless you have been a vegetarian for years and are extremely adept at using substitute foods and understand their nutritional values. Common sense demands, that if you are to regain good health, you must have a well balanced diet planned from within the range of foods you are permitted.

Do make sure the meat you select is from an organic source. Fish and rabbit is relatively uncontaminated, and free range chickens are now quite easy to obtain. It's just the red meats you need to be cautious with.

I do not recommend veganism at all. It is far too restrictive to allow for a healthy balance. The foods left to you are not adequate for the nutritional needs of the body because of modern food farming techniques. Whatever you do, make certain you don't have the same foods day in day out. Firstly you will be restricting your vitamin and mineral intake, and secondly you could breed further allergies by repetitive eating, therefore, keep having a good variety.

When you add fruit into the diet at the end of the first month, don't eat it at the same meal as you have meat. Why? Because meat takes 12 hours to go through the alimentary tract, while fruit only takes about 20-30 minutes. This means that the fruit could get trapped behind the meat in your system and ferment, something you should avoid at all costs. So eat your fruit on an empty stomach, between meals and always in the morning.

Well now, I think that's all the rules.

"Eat yourself well"

DOCTORS - dealing with them

It is a great pity there is need to include this heading. There should be nothing of import to say on the subject. Ideally, your doctor should be your confidant and friend, ready to do anything he/she can to restore you to good health. Unfortunately, in today's world, this is rarely the case. Some of the stories I have been told in the clinic by clients about their experiences have been truly horrific.

Many people are in awe of their doctor and I can't help wondering if medical colleges include a special, obligatory course on "How to intimidate your patient." Many of them have a special knack of making you feel you really have no right to be consulting them, but since you're here, get on with it and don't waste time. O.K. So they are busy. Maybe you would be too if you hadn't spent the last 2 hours waiting because the appointment system fouled up. When you are finally summoned, you drag out your list of symptoms and things you want to ask. You have to write it all down in case you are hurried so much you forget something crucial and and have to go to the end of the queue and lose another day and more time and money. Who pays these people anyway?

Doctors don't often look up. They are busy either computing notes on the patient who just left, or prescribing for you on the basis of information from your last visit. It will be either antibiotics, steroids, hormones or tranquilizers. The odd pain killer may be thrown in. You decide you have had enough of these fruitless trips to the surgery and make a real effort to grab attention. You say you suspect you have a yeast infection. You are rewarded with a cynical smile and, "Rubbish! No such thing, you don't want to believe what you read in the papers." With just a cursory glance, you are referred to a psychiatrist.

At the time of writing I am treating a 15 year old girl whose mother has been told by her doctor she has anorexia nervosa, (although the symptoms are more indicative of bulimia) and unless she takes tranquilizers and sees a psychiatrist, she will die and her mother will be responsible for her death. No dietary advice has been given, no compassion shown. The reasons for her being unable to keep her meals down have been brushed aside as imagination. When they came to me, both mother and daughter were in a terribly nervous state, not because of illness, but because of the way they had been treated. The girl has Candida and it will be under control in 4 to 6 months. Already, after just one week of treatment she has begun to eat well, stopped being sick and has put on a couple of pounds.

Another client constantly refers to her doctor as **GOD** because she says, he behaves as though he is God.

Those are the bad stories, but some doctors do listen and are becoming increasingly aware of the Candida / M.E. situation. Some have written or phoned for information asking how best to provide the needed supplements. Whilst progress was made in Britain for supplements to be made available on the National Health Service, when I first compiled this book in 1993, changes in government policy have reversed the situation and at the time of revising information nothing can be prescribed. However, some doctors have come to recognize the dangers of prescribing antibiotics for every cough and sniffle. These are the ones who have kept themselves up to date with current findings and who have not forgotten the oath they took when they qualified. You may be surprised to learn how it reads:-

The Hippocratic Oath

"I will follow that system or regimen which, according to my ability and judgment, I consider to be *for the benefit of my patients, and abstain from whatever is deleterious and mischievous.* I will give no deadly medicine to anyone if asked nor suggest any such counsel, and in like manner I will not give to a woman the means to produce an abortion. Whenever I go into a house, I will go for the benefit of the sick and will abstain from every voluntary act of mischief and corruption, and further, from the seduction of females or males, whether freemen or slaves. Whatever, in connection with my professional practice, I see or hear which ought not to be spoken abroad, I will keep secret. So long as I continue to carry out this oath unviolated, may it be granted to me to enjoy life and the practice of the art, respected by all men in all times, but should I violate this oath, may the reverse be my lot."

Hippocrates the originator of that oath and the father of medicine, also taught his students, "First do no harm." Modern medicine seems to have changed the rules.

If you do have a doctor who really is interested in helping you, you are indeed blessed, and he will give you all the support within his power. Please be cautious though because some, believing they are helping, prescribe antifungal drugs such as Nystatin, Nystan, Nisorol, Fungalin, Fluconazole, Flucytosine, Diflucan, Sporanox, etc. Whilst it is true, these drugs do kill off the fungal infections initially, in the long term they can actually predispose the formation of stronger strains of yeast growth and increase the number of colonies formed later. They are called polyene antibiotics. The only positive way to regain good health is naturally.

If the doctor insists on writing a prescription for you, and you live in Britain, you can ask the chemist if you can look at the British National Formulary to check on the side effects, cautions and contra indications of the prescribed drug. Other countries may have similar systems. It does no harm to ask. When you are fully informed of the possible consequences of taking the medication, you may decide the side effects may prove worse than the symptoms you are currently experiencing.

Whatever your doctor's attitude and approach, you should remember, in the social structure under which we live, we are dependent upon our doctor for health care and hospitalization for illnesses and accidents unrelated to Candida and M.E. If we have a heart attack, break a leg, or need emergency treatment requiring expensive equipment only available in hospitals, then we have to be referred by our doctor. So we need to keep an amicable relationship with him/her. Don't be antagonistic. If you can't agree, drop the subject. Accept his prescriptions but don't necessarily have them processed. You are the custodian of your body and you do not have to take advice you consider unacceptable. *Be brave, be wise. Keep your options open.* Above all, don't be intimidated into taking drugs that could result in making you worse.

"Defend yourself, but with respect"

EATING NORMALLY AGAIN

People often ask me if eating normally again will ever be possible for them. There is no straight answer. You must consider why you became ill in the first place. Often the cause of Candida or M.E. cannot be traced back to the use of antibiotics, hormones or steroids, although they are the most usual. It may be you have been affected by hereditary illness, environmental pollutants, a mouldy dwelling or a number of other factors, but by far the most likely other cause of illness can be traced back to the over use of cane sugar and bread in the western diet. As children, sweets are often given as treats or as a reward system. Children's parties are designed around sugar covered cakes, chocolate treats and a host of other highly sweetened "goodies." We grow up associating sugary foods with the good times in life. This conditions us to expect sweet foods when we need reassurance that things are going well for us. Bread has been imposed on our subconscious in a similar way. "The staff of life" makes a quick sandwich. It is a cheap meal to satisfy us until a proper meal time. Of themselves neither food is all bad. It is the constant and repetitive use of them that's the root of the trouble.

So when I am asked that question, I counter with, "What is normal?" 'Normal' must be a diet low in sugar, with a proper balance and variety of natural, unrefined, additive free foods to supply the body with adequate nutrients to ensure good health. Always continue to select organic vegetables and fruit whenever possible. If not, make sure to peel everything. Once you have become used to quality organic meat, you will never want to return to eating the tasteless variety others tolerate and call 'normal'.

When your health is restored, then you can enjoy the occasional flight of fancy into the realms of 'goodies', but remember, they are not normal. If indulged in repeatedly, they will lead you back to all the old problems.

"Eat well, but eat with care"

EATING OUT

Eating out can be one of life's great pleasures. Unfortunately for Candida, M.E and allergy sufferers it is fraught with danger and misery. The danger of eating something forbidden on the diet, is that it may give you an allergic reaction for a week or more. It may also make you miserable watching others enjoy foods you can't have.

You have two choices, (1) don't go, or (2) go, but think positively. Face up to the problems and *advise those you plan to eat with of your difficulty.* It helps them to understand your behaviour.

Now sit down and make a list of foods you **CAN** have. If you know where you are going to eat, speak to the chef, tell him / her of your problem and give them a list of 'safe foods', asking them to prepare a meal for you from the list. You will be delighted with your meal. Cooks love a challenge and will take pleasure in pleasing you.

If you don't know where you will dine, just try handing your list, with a short explanation written on the top, to the person waiting at table as you enter. They will either help you to select suitable dishes from the menu, or ask the chef to prepare something especially for you. You will be pleasantly surprised how helpful everyone can be if you make it brief and easy for them. It is only when you tell them what you can't have you will experience difficulties.

Perhaps you will be eating at a friend's home. Phone and give them your list well in advance, to give them thinking time. They will usually be happy to comply with your request. If they won't they aren't real friends.

Day trip eating out is not difficult. Salads are plentiful but watch the dressings. Jacket potatoes are popular, fish and chips are everywhere (leave the batter) and kebabs are filling and delicious. There is great variety to choose from. Your companions may finish up envying you.

"Bon appetite"

ELECTROMAGNETISM and M.E.

Practitioners who treat M.E. will agree, some patients respond well to probiotic treatment, making steady progress back to health. Others though, improve initially and then reach a plateau beyond which they cannot go. This is difficult to understand until you learn about the effects of electromagnetism on the brain.

Simply put, there is a small section in the centre of the two halves of the brain called the thalamus. It is the central control for all our bodily impulses and is capable of sending thousands of different signals, like radio waves, into all parts of the body to govern cell activity.

Underneath the thalamus lies the hypothalamus which works as a control for the pituitary gland, switching us off for sleep. There are different phases of sleep throughout the night. One of them is known as 'paradoxical sleep'. This is the time when messages are sent from the brain to damaged body cells to be repaired. Electromagnetism can interfere with this process by blocking hypothalamus activity.

To illustrate, it can be likened to what happens when a 'ham' radio operator broadcasts on the same frequency as another station, the wavelength is blocked.

The question is, what happens if the hypothalamus malfunctions? Not only is our sleep pattern disturbed, but also cells do not receive the commands from the brain to restore and correct health problems.

What causes this interference? The answer is, the world of technological advancement. All of us are subjected to 'electric smog' to some extent. If not in our workplace, then possibly in our homes because of using so many electrical appliances.

It is impossible to escape the increasing use of televisions, radios, radar, commercial and weather satellites, overhead power cables on pylons, microwave ovens, computers, photocopiers, hairdryers, vacuum cleaners etc. All of these items give off electromagnetic energy capable of blocking our 'brain waves'.

Knowing how water is a conductor for electricity, it then becomes easy to understand how people who live close to or above underground waterways can be adversely affected by 'bad' energy for many hours each day. Even culvert sewage pipes could be an ecological hazard.

We are particularly vulnerable while we sleep because we remain in one spot for a number of hours. If our bed is in the direct path of electromagnetic energy our health may be severely damaged.

When M.E. sufferers are unable to make progress it would be wise to look at the electromagnetic picture in their environment and remove the individual from as much 'smog' as possible. They will then make improvement.

Because this hazard is invisible, it is often forgotten or ignored.

" Don't fail to be switched on to the presence and affects of electromagnetism"

ENCOURAGEMENT

Oh! How we all need encouragement, even when we are well. How much more so when we are ill, feeling low and on a restrictive diet. There will be days when you feel you simply can't go on. You will be sick of being told you are some kind of crank, sick of the pill popping, sick of all the criticism and above all sick of the ****** diet.

Tired of reading interminable labels, the family are driving you crazy and you feel like bursting into tears and pigging out on the entire contents of the fridge, the cupboard and the corner shop. You just can't see all the effort you have made has made any difference at all.

Would it help you to know other sufferers have days when they feel exactly as you do? These are the days when you need all the encouragement you can get. If you have followed my suggestion to note down all your symptoms before starting the programme, now is the time to read through it. You will be pleasantly surprised when you see how many of the initial symptoms have gone. This knowledge should cheer you a bit and strengthen your resolve to keep going.

Why not phone your practitioner and say how you feel, there should be words to encourage you to keep going, maybe they can tell you of others who stayed the course and are now fit and well.

You could try reading the letters section of this book and see how others have recovered by seeing it through. Think of how long you have been on the confounded diet, all the money you have spent on supplements, what willpower you have shown. Think of the weight loss or gain, (depending on which way you are going) if you continue. Think of the person who saw you the other day who told you how much better you looked and how different. Encourage yourself. Pat yourself on the back and think how good life will be when you have finally beaten this thing. ***Whatever you do, don't give up now, you have done so well***. If you break the rules now, you will have to begin all over again at a later date, or be ill for the rest of your life. Cheer up, phone a friend and have a natter about something other than your health. Have a couple of yeast free crackers, some feta cheese and a hot drink and count your blessings. It could be worse, at least you know what to do to get well, some people have no hope for their illnesses.

Comfort yourself with the knowledge there is at least one person who knows how you feel, and cares.... Me! And I am sure there are many more who know and love you. Just like the ones who bring their loved ones to me for help. They spend time, money and effort to show they care. These are the ones who daily have to stand by watching as a friend or family member goes through the pain, weakness and sheer indignities those who suffer with Candida and M.E. know so well.

These are also the ones who often try to help financially and practically. They shop, cook, clean, drive and do many other chores. Is it any wonder they sometimes forget how to laugh? Their lives too can become devoid of joy. Try to be an encouragement to one another. Try to see the funny side of things and laugh together. If you can share the problems you will strengthen, not only the bond between you, but the spirit to go on, in both of you.

"Chin up and soldier on"

ENERGY AND EXERCISE

Lack of energy is a major symptom in both Candida and M.E. It is important to conserve it at all costs. When the body is fighting illness it needs every iota of energy to convert into healing power, so it must not be wasted on non essentials.

Try to find ways of cutting down on energy expenditure in any way you can and enlist the help of others whenever possible. Here are a few suggestions.

For instance, looking after your hair can take major effort if it is long. Why not change to a good, short cut style that simply needs washing, combing into place and leaving to dry naturally. Clothes that slip over your head can eliminate the need to struggle with zips and buttons. Slip on shoes. Elastic waistbands.

If you are a mother, enlist the aid of the children to vacuum, dust and tidy. Encourage them to go shopping for you, or prepare vegetables for dinner and afterward to take their turn at washing up. It is not only helpful to you, but will teach them about life.

Visitors often ask if there is anything they can do to help. Don't tell them you can manage, find something for them to do for you. You will conserve your strength and they will feel useful and be glad they came. It might even encourage them to come again when they realize they can be helpful instead of sitting trying to make small talk.

Don't try to exercise while you are low. When you begin to improve, the tendency is to overdo it. Don't be tempted too soon, you will only become exhausted and make yourself ill again. Wait! The day will come when you can do things without ill effects, but that day will not be the first time you think of trying. Give your system time to re-establish itself and build up something in reserve. When you finally do start, take it really slow and easy.

Something more should be taken into account when human energy is being considered. Energy is the fuel of life. When God made

71

man, He made him from the dust of the ground, then the Bible says "He, breathed into him the Breath of Life... and man came to be a living soul." Breath = air, so our life force is fueled by our intake of oxygen and the 'dust' or food we eat.

If your breathing is restricted, or air quality is poor, or your diet is inadequate, your energy levels will be low. While your exercise is limited, make sure you breathe deeply and be vigilant about the quality of your air space. Don't allow smokers in your presence and don't smoke yourself. If air quality is poor in your area, due to high pollution levels, you might consider installing air conditioning in your home, or even moving.

Similar care must be taken when selecting food. Buy the best. Organic and free range produce may cost more but the benefits are well worth the extra expenditure. Also, because refining removes roughage it reduces the bulk of the foods. Buying and eating unrefined foods means you will eat less, becoming satisfied more easily, so you won't need to buy so much. It eventually balances itself out. When you purchase quality foods you buy extra energy.

Lastly we should pay attention to the proper balance of energy throughout the human frame. Acupuncture, Shiatsu, Applied Kinesiology, Reflexology and associated therapies can do much to ensure good energy distribution via the meridians and energy channels known to eastern medicine for thousands of years. A good practitioner or masseur will be able to raise your energy levels, thereby speeding up recovery. A warning here, these therapies are very helpful but will not alone, control your Candida, M.E. or allergies. *They support, not replace the diet and supplement programme.*

"Rest results in Bouncing Back"

EXPECTATIONS OF RECOVERY

Knowing what to expect, right from the start, can be reassuring in any situation. It is vitally important for the Candida, M.E. and allergy sufferer. The first thing everyone asks is "How long will it take to be well again?" The answer depends on a number of things. How long have you been ill? Has it been lurking since childhood as ear infections, sore throats, nappy rash as a baby? Or has it been a relatively new development? Next, how old are you? How many years has the condition gone unnoticed and untreated?

If you are still young and have only recently become ill, you have a good chance of being well in around six months, but if you are older and it has been of long duration, then you must be prepared for anything up to three years before you really are better. This doesn't mean you will continue feeling as ill as you do now for all that time, you will be making slow progress back to good health.

Sometimes it is hard to see the changes for the better, because you are too close to the problem. Progress can be likened to the growth of a child. Mum sees the child everyday and is only aware of changes when his trousers become short or his shoes cramp his toes, but a visiting relative who hasn't seen the child for some time will exclaim, "My, how you've grown." Friends may notice and tell you how much better you look.

Another important factor will be how faithfully you keep to the regime. If you constantly break the diet or neglect to take your supplements it will take you longer to get well, that is, if you ever achieve it at all. Just to let you know how devastating a little sugar can be I shall quote from an article in Biologist magazine entitled "Candida albicans" by Michael F. Tuite. (1990) 37 (3) "A single cell of Candida albicans can multiply up to 100,000,000 in 48 hours when fed with a teaspoonful of sugar."

I cannot stress enough how important it is for you to be consistent with the supplements. Your body must be given the building blocks needed if it is to repair itself.

So, to a certain extent **YOU** determine the length of time it will take you to be well. Don't be despondent if you think you aren't making progress. The very nature of the illness means it is going to be two steps forward and one back. If you made a list of symptoms at the start, go through them again and you will see how many of them have gone. This will encourage you to plod on.

"Patience pays off"

FAMILY AND FRIENDS

Our nearest and dearest should be our greatest source of support whilst we are unwell, often they are. Sadly though, sometimes they add to our problems. Usually because they fail to understand the nature of our illness and believe our diet is too restrictive. After all they are able to consume large quantities of 'junk' food with no ill effects. So they can't see why you are unable to do the same.

It could be because they have never been ill and have no concept of what it is like to hurt all over. Or sometimes they are just plain nasty, thoughtless and selfish, and all they can worry about is how your incapacity is affecting them.

Occasionally they may put pressure on you to take the drugs the doctor prescribes because in their opinion the doctor must know best, or alternative treatments will cost money which they resent parting with. They may even call it a 'waste'.

Often the long term nature of the illness, and it's treatment is hard for them to understand or accept because they have become accustomed to the 'instant' results modern medicine usually appears to produce.

All these situations will be hard for you to cope with. If you were well you might be able to deal with the hassle, but while you are ill it can be soul destroying. It could lead to you giving up your treatment, breaking the diet, or trying drug therapies, even though you know they don't work. ***Don't let them do it to you.*** You have a right to good health and this is the way back to it so ***keep going no matter what they say.***

"Love them but ignore them"

FASTING

This is a wonderful way of helping yourself to feel better. Fast! (if you'll pardon the pun). It is the finest way to encourage your body to shed its toxic load. In today's world, even the best quality foods cannot be guaranteed totally free from contamination because the earth, air and water on this planet are so polluted. We in the western world are guilty of eating far more than our bodies actually need to sustain life and energy. Consequently we have diet related health problems. When we stop eating for a while we give our body an opportunity for a 'spring clean'. There are so many advantages to fasting.

The most common fear about fasting is that going without food will damage your health. The only people who should not fast are diabetics, those with malnutrition, and people who are severely mentally and physically exhausted after surgery. It would also be unwise for those in the advanced stages of cancer, tuberculosis or similar illnesses that cause interminable weight loss, although it has been reported as beneficial even then. The rest of us can only do ourselves good by fasting. Particularly Candida and M.E. sufferers. It also brings the added benefit of a total respite from food allergy reactions.

People often express worry they will die after only a few days deprived of food. This simply isn't true. You cannot survive for more than a few days without water, so if you do fast, make sure you drink between 3.5 and 4.5 litres (6 and 8 pints) daily, however, you can survive for several weeks without food with no ill effects whatsoever.

All you need to do to begin a fast is to refuse a meal. Hey presto! You have begun! At first you will feel hungry but overcome this by drinking spring or filtered water. Hunger diminishes in a couple of days. It is surprising how quickly your body can adjust to not eating. The first two days are the worst. You may have headaches and withdrawal symptoms, especially from tea, coffee and sugar. By day three most people just feel tired, so plan a lazy, quiet day. On days four and five you will hardly recognize yourself. More energy and vitality. Hair and eyes shining and feeling positive about everything.

Make sure your bowels continue to open regularly. If they don't, give them some help with Glauber salts or an enema. You must be sure to eliminate properly.

The advantages are greatest for Candida sufferers, because, not only are you ridding your body of toxins but you are also starving the Candida to death. M.E. sufferers often find their greatest advantage is the loss of muscular pain and weakness and both groups find their digestion improves after the 'holiday'.

Do not take supplements whilst you are fasting, they are food.

More benefits, you are not only saving on food bills but also on supplements. The longer you continue, the greater the benefits. Some, after the recommended five days, choose to continue longer because it is easier than they imagined. I would consider four weeks to be the absolute maximum.

I should make it clear I am talking about *total fasting*. Some suggest taking vegetable or fruit juices but this will render the procedure invalid because you will be continuing to consume fructose (fruit sugar) which in turn will feed candidiasis.

If you do fast, don't be tempted to 'just have a little nibble'. It will start your taste buds and digestive juices off and bring back your hunger pangs. This makes it hard to continue.

The best time to choose is just before you start the programme, you then retrain your taste buds to accept the different diet. When you have had nothing, everything tastes good.

Just one week could change your health, Why not have a go? You have nothing to lose.

"Get in the 'fast' lane"

FLATULANCE

This is a subject some people find most embarrassing whilst others find it highly amusing. Either way we are all better off without it. To those with any kind of gut disorder it can be source of continual irritation. What can be done about it?

First examine your diet. Are you consuming large quantities of pulses, or onions? To quote one of my instructors, "They are extremely farty." If you are using them regularly, try cutting them out for a few days and see if you improve. Some people find red meat causes rumblings and wind because it lays in the digestive tract for so long. Try just having chicken and fish to see if it helps. You could also experiment with your bacteria powder. Maybe your system needs a little more or perhaps less than you are taking each day.

Only try one solution at a time, otherwise you won't know which is working for you. Something else to consider is, your colon is quite likely to be corroded with years of impacted faecal debris. The treatment programme is stirring things up for a grand spring clean. While this is happening, all sorts of gases will be produced, but as your bowels become clean and normalize, the problem will solve itself.

Meanwhile learn to say, "Whoops, pardon me" and flash everyone your most devastating smiles. Failing that, blame the dog.

"I hope this heading won't cause a stink"

FOLLOWING THROUGH

When you have finally completed your course of treatment and you are feeling better, that's the time to take stock of what you intend to do about your health for the rest of your life.

Now you are well, you should give thought to trying to stay that way, especially as you know your body has a tendency to succumb to this very serious condition. You are in possession of knowledge about food and the environment you didn't have before. You are informed about ecological pollutants, and have first hand experience of how sick this world has become. Will you revert to the way of life you had before? Or will you learn from your experience and be more cautious in future? Take care of yourself more, watching for signs of decline in your health. If it happens, do something fast, before the problem gets a firm hold again.

When clients leave the clinic 'well' after a course of treatment, I urge them to be sensible about eating habits. Introduce foods back into your diet little by little with only the occasional 'special treat'. Don't go back to repetitive bread or dairy produce. The world around hasn't changed for the better. It is probably getting worse as you read this. The fact you are now well proves the diet you have been following is a good one, so why not stick to it most of the time, with just an occasional 'splurge.'

Another thing you have learned is that your body responds well to the supplements you have been taking, so why not continue at a reduced dosage to give your immune system time to become really strong again. You can stop the anti-fungal product, it has done its work, but I recommend continuing the vitamins and bacteria at half dose, slowly reducing to a third. Keep on until you are absolutely sure you have attained full recovery of your immune defenses. Although you have triumphed over the initial invasion, you should be aware, it takes approximately three years for the immune system to fully recover. Do follow through.

"Never let your defenses down"

FOOD

Of necessity, the selection, preparation and consumption of food must have your earnest attention.

If your eating habits are faulty, your attempts to achieve good health will fail. You need to find sources of organic, free range foods, devoid of additives and preservatives. For town dwellers it's easy. The Superstores are increasingly catering for these needs. They usually stock goat and sheep milk, yoghurt and cheeses, non dairy margarine, a selection of organically grown vegetables, free range chickens and eggs, fish and vegetarian cheeses. Some stock organic soups and tinned fish in brine. Tinned fruit without added sugar and organic rice and flours are also on the shelves. Fructose is also readily available.

The best thing to do is list the foods you want, then search the shops, noting down where you found the foods you wanted. Read all the labels carefully. If you don't have the energy to shop, why not phone the stores with your list and ask if they have the items you need. When you know if things are available, you only have to make one journey. Some stores will deliver.

If you live in the country, you may have the advantage of having fresh organic produce from a farm, or even be able to grow your own. Often country folk keep chickens and sell eggs and goat milk from their homes.

There are also companies prepared to send specialist foods by post. Order either by telephone or through the internet. There are some names in this book under 'Useful addresses'. It is easy to become downhearted about a restricted diet, but more and more quality foods are now becoming available in all sorts of ways.

"Don't get fed up"

FRUIT

The instructions for your diet will say no fruit for the first month of your programme. This is because of the high fructose (fruit sugar) content of fruit. To initially starve out the Candida, anything with even a suspicion of sweetness must be excluded. This doesn't mean you can't eat fruit for the whole time you are on the programme, but it is wise to *introduce it very slowly, after the first four weeks without.*

Just have one piece per day to begin with, making it a different kind of fruit each day. For example, an apple on Monday, a pear on Tuesday, an orange on Wednesday, mango on Thursday, banana on Friday and so on, rotating the fruit to allow a variety of fructose levels for your body to handle from day to day.

From the fourth month of treatment, if the sufferer is making good progress and feels well, I allow some dried fruit to be added to cooking, so long as it is carefully selected to avoid moulds when bought.

As you reintroduce fruit, listen to your body, if worsening of symptoms occur, stop eating it immediately, wait for another month before trying again. You don't want to destroy the good you have achieved.

"Be cautious about getting 'fruity'"

GENETICS

One thing is for sure, we are all the result of our ancestors health, or lack of it. Just as surely as we inherit brown or blue eyes, dark or fair hair or black or white skin, we are either the recipients of a strong or weak constitution or something in between depending on what our forefathers had to hand down to us.

If your parents passed a weak immune system on to you, then it is unlikely you will ever be able to change to being totally robust, but over a period of time, with sensible living and eating habits, you will be able to improve and strengthen what you have, in order to give you some added protection against disease. You may even be able to pass on an improved standard of life to any offspring you may have. Surely that thought should spur us on to try to attain optimum health for ourselves? After all we all want the best for our children.

Many of the health problems we assume are inherited, are really acquired. Think about it. Who taught us to eat? To eat what? What kind of environment were we born into? What standard of accommodation do we tolerate? Which form of medication was inflicted upon us before we were old enough to choose? All these factors and many more have had an effect on the kind of health we are experiencing now.

We are all the sum total of our lifestyle up to this moment, but we can change many of these factors for the better to gain an improvement for ourselves When we have made a real effort to do this, then the health problems we are left with will be truly genetic ones.

"Don't blame your D.N.A. until you're sure
it is really at fault"

GOOD HEALTH

What is it? How do we know when we have it? When you have been ill for a long time, it is easy to forget how it feels to be well.

Let's just analyze how we should be. We ought to wake with a sense of quiet apprehension about what our day will bring, and a desire to achieve something within the day. A feeling of gladness at being alive. The kind of weather outside should not affect us from the standpoint of our health. We simply select the appropriate clothing according to the activities in which we intend to participate. It should be a pleasure to rise from our bed and our minds should hold an eager anticipation of what the day will bring. With a twinkle in our eye, a lilt in our step, our skin clear and our hair shining, an aura of well being radiating from us.

It ought to be easy to be pleasant to our family and those with whom we come in contact throughout the day. Capable of taking problems in our stride, attaining a full day's activity, be it work or play, at the end, feeling comfortably tired and ready to relax, we should then fall into a refreshing, sound sleep.

That is the ideal. Of course there will be circumstances to take into account for you as an individual, such as hereditary problems, or previously sustained injuries, but generally you ought to feel, look and behave well if you are in good health.

You will know when you are really well when you come to the end of a day and realize you didn't have to think about your health and were totally unconscious of your body all day. That is what you are trying to attain. Keep taking the tablets and watching your diet, and one day soon you will achieve it.

"Good health 'Sparkles'"

HALITOSIS - Bad Breath

Bad breath can be a very real worry for sufferers in the early stages of treatment for Candida and M.E. and also an indication of allergic reactions to some foods. It is due to a number of alimentary problems, such as lack of absorption and fermentation. The most usual cause is a lack of 'friendly flora'. As the programme progresses and the bacteria is reestablished the problem resolves itself.

It can also be due to impacted faeces in the intestines causing putrefaction in the gut. This can only be put right by cleansing the system and sometimes takes considerable time to achieve. Cleansing programmes are available using psyllium husks, herbs and L. Acidophilus. Naturally, if digestion is poor, this too can lead to unpleasant breath, as will eating foods that don't agree with us.

Many complain about the garlic they take whilst on the course. Others often complain to them about it. I know in some circles it is considered anti social, but with travel abroad for holidays becoming more popular, the cuisine of other countries is becoming more acceptable. For our health's sake we need it. If a family member is the complainant sneak some into their food and they won't be able to smell yours.

Garlic is one of the most ancient healers known to man and is an essential part of your programme. If you really can't tolerate the smell, then munch parsley, or drink parsley tea. This will neutralize the aroma.

Whatever you do, make sure you keep taking the garlic.

"Smell and become well"

HERXHEIMER REACTION

This is a term used by practitioners to describe what happens when Candida treatment causes the parasite to 'die off'. The dead organisms then become toxic waste in the system and contaminate the blood stream causing a variety of distressing symptoms.

Some think they are having a bad attack of 'flu' as the body aches miserably all over. Others have experienced an exaggerated reaction combining most, if not all of the symptoms they have had over a period of years. Most feel totally wretched while this is happening and some become extremely frightened.

Amongst the most distressing of the reactions can be, abdominal bloating, excessive flatulence, outbreaks of mouth ulcers or abscess, ear aches, depression and thrush or other vaginal discharges in women. A period of impotence is not uncommon in men and a huge variety of other symptoms can occur, some of which may be peculiar to you alone.

One young woman who attended the clinic had a herpes sore that stretched from midway up her neck to just below her eyes and round to both ears. It lasted three weeks and both her mother and I feared she would be scarred for life. She wasn't, and what is more, the acne she had been plagued with for many years, and was one of the symptoms she worried about most, has completely gone. The last I heard she was fitter than she had ever been, had married and had given birth to her second healthy child. She had been a Spina-Bifida baby born with club feet and had been subjected to more operations and chemical medication than any other four people I have ever treated put together. All the residue had to find a way out of her system.

Hers was an extreme reaction and her situation was unique so don't be frightened into thinking it is the same for everyone. You are an individual and your reactions if any will be uniquely your own. If you have them, you can make them bearable by taking extra care of yourself for a few days until they pass. Rest and give your body the best opportunity to readjust and clear out the toxins.

Drink plenty of spring or filtered water to flush your system and if you can find someone qualified to do it, have a deep, lymphatic drainage massage, using aromatherapy oils and acupressure techniques. This will clear the toxins from the body quickly and make you feel better sooner than if you left it to happen on its own.

Remember *it will pass* and when it does, you will feel better than you have in ages. Also you will be well on the road to complete recovery.

Whatever you do,

DON'T BE TEMPTED TO TAKE ANTIBIOTICS OR ANY CHEMICALLY PREPARED MEDICATION.

This reaction is your body's way of trying to rid itself of all the accumulation of them you have taken in the past. If you do take them again, you will most certainly undo all the good you have achieved up to this stage.

"Give your body the opportunity to correct itself naturally"

HOMEOPATHIC TREATMENT

Many people think if a treatment is alternative, it must come under the heading of homeopathy. This is not true. Homeopathy is a very separate and exact science. Derived from the Greek word homoios, meaning 'like'. Homeopathy is the practice of treating like with like. This means treating the sick person with a substance which produces similar symptoms to those already being displayed.

It sees the symptoms as the body's reaction against illness as it attempts to overcome it, rather than the current orthodox view, that symptoms are manifestations of the illness. In seeking to stimulate the symptoms it attempts to help the body rid itself of the disease. Dorlands medical dictionary says, "a system of therapeutics based on the administration of minute doses of drugs which are capable of producing in healthy persons symptoms like those of the disease treated."

Though being valuable in most illnesses, it is limited in the treatment of Candida and M.E. In both conditions the immune system is severely depressed, so is incapable of responding in the same way. First, immune responses must be restored with the diet and supplements.

Homeopathy may however prove useful in treating minor problems whilst you are struggling to improve your overall condition. Some M.E. sufferers have found it helpful in alleviating insomnia or feelings of despair.

Bach flower remedies can be of great help in improving the psychological outlook. They are easily available at most health shops, or a good practitioner will make one to fit your specific needs.

"similia similibus curentur"
"like cures like"

HYPERACTIVITY

This is not often a problem for adults suffering from Candida and it is most certainly not a symptom of M.E. Quite the reverse. It can however be a sign of allergic reaction and it deserves inclusion in this book because it is one of the earliest indications of a Candida overgrowth.

In an adult it may be assumed they are just highly energetic people, but if carefully observed it will be noticeable that the individual finds it impossible to be still even for a short period. They hurry everything. Trotting along instead of walking, legs twitching and fingers drumming when they sit or lay. They often complain of a bubbly feeling in their tummy. They talk so fast, you don't have time to take a breath to reply. You feel tired just watching them, or having them around. They don't feel ill as yet, but if this is allowed to continue they soon will.

Their constant state of activity is derived from yeast starting to ferment in their gut, a bit like alcoholic indulgence, it makes you feel good at first but as time progresses you begin to feel sluggish, your legs give out and you fall into a state of inertia. The same thing happens to a hyperactive individual. They are fermenting inside, but eventually the Candida overgrowth will gain a hold and slow them down. Or they will be diagnosed as M.E. victims when their bodies become so over tired they can't cope anymore.

Allergy sufferers are prone to having a hyperactive period after eating certain foods, ingesting or being in the vicinity of chemicals that affect them. This can be a sign that Candida has become a problem, but not always.

Children are particularly prone to hyperactivity. It will be the start of a lifetime of poor health unless treated before puberty. If you have a hyperactive child, get help for them now. (See heading Kids and Candida.)

" Hype is not healthy"

IMMUNE SYSTEM, INFLAMMATORY BOWEL DISEASE and I.B.S.

This heading is a study on its own and deserves a whole book to explain its implications. All three conditions named above have the same root cause. Initially, an overgrowth of Candida albicans.

There are a variety of names given to the devastation Candida causes in the human gut. It depends on where the problem arises. You are probably familiar with some of the medical terms used. By far the most common is I.B.S. Short for irritable bowel syndrome. This diagnosis is usually only the beginning of a downward spiral as the bowel becomes more and more distressed. These are some others you may be familiar with, diverticulitis, ulcerative and mucous colitis and Crohn's disease. They are all the start of what are known as auto-immune disorders

In order to explain the connection between these bowel conditions and Candida albicans, I need first to describe the way the immune system works.

The immune system can be likened to a large army of cells, all with different tasks to do to defend the human body against invasion by disease. The front line of this army are called Lymphocytes. These are white blood cells. Under normal conditions they produce antibodies. Antibodies are generated in response to the invasion of foreign substances, which it is their job to neutralize, thus producing immunity against infection. Not all Lymphocytes are the same. Some, called T cells, are the 'generals' of the army. They are the ones who give the orders and plan the site of attack. They have the responsibility for sending out B cells and their antibodies to attack hostile intruders. T cells also programme the Lymphocytes not to turn on and attack self, or the good, friendly bacteria so vital to health. Each Lymphocyte is programmed to look after a certain part of the body, or body system to keep everything in proper order.

The above is how it all was designed to work, but in 'auto

89

immune' diseases, the 'generals', or T cells become disorientated and give the wrong orders to certain parts of the body. The result is, instead of protecting their part, the B killers turn and attack what they are meant to defend.

If the site of the battle is the bowel, then the above illnesses develop, because natural defences are destroyed.

It is at this point that invasion by parasites occurs and Candida albicans is one of the first to grow out of control as the immune system is progressively weakened by the absence of 'friendly flora'

Practically everyone who suffers with an inflammatory bowel disease also has a severe Candida albicans overgrowth. Drugs may hold back the inflammation for a while, but more often, they simply encourage formation of more candidiasis. They never solve the real cause, the depleted immune system. Only a natural programme can do it, comprising of a revised diet, vitamin and mineral supplementation and reestablishment of bacteria as suggested in this book. In really serious, life threatening cases, bacterial implantation has been used both orally and rectally with impressive results.

In the case of M.E. the immune system turns and attacks other sites in the body. These sites under attack vary from person to person, that is why there can be such a diversity of symptoms. (See heading M.E. What is it?)

"A clean colon means improved health"

90

IMPOTENCE

This is a common problem for men who contract M.E. or Candida and believe me it is, for them, the symptom giving them most concern. Their very manhood is at stake, or so it seems to them.

Please fella's, let me reassure you, *you will do it again,* maybe not tomorrow, but in the not too distant future. You may think you are the only man on earth who can't perform. *That isn't so.*

If we are to believe the media and the world of advertising, everyone does it at least three times a night and wakes up panting for more. The true facts are, even people in regular relationships don't do it that much, some married couples confessed to only being bothered with it a couple of times a year. Most of the sex that is said to go on is in the head, or an exaggerated boast.

The first step to restoring sex drive is to stop worrying about it and give your attention to the cause of the problem, the Candida or M.E. If you keep strictly to your programme, you will soon be better and it won't be long before things begin to 'look up'.

Sex starts in the mind, then the body follows through. When your mind stops making you feel inadequate and your body is free of the lethargy and fatigue you have been experiencing you will soon recover your zing... and....

*"It won't be long before you
are well away again"*

JOURNEYS

The thought of traveling any distance when you are ill can fill you with trepidation. You may decide you could not possibly cope with the problems entailed and deprive yourself of an opportunity to meet with friends, or see sights to lift your spirits and take you out of the same four walls. Maybe the decision not to go is right, but sometimes, with a little thought and forward planning, you could enjoy an outing or a holiday and it would do you good.

First, you should plan your physical comfort en-route. If you are going by car, have the back seat equipped with a pillow and blanket in order to be able to take a nap in comfort when you want to. If you are traveling by plane, phone the airline and explain you have bowel problems and muscular weakness, they can arrange for you to occupy the seat on the aisle, directly next to the toilet where there is extra leg room. The air hostesses are always happy to find you a pillow and blanket to make you snug.

You can also inform them of your dietary needs, then they can ensure your in-flight meals will be appropriate to your needs. You can also ask for a wheelchair to be supplied to save you the long walk to the plane.

Your bacteria powder must go with you and needs to be kept at the right temperature. This can be done by placing it, complete with the amber jar and straight from the refrigerator, into a wide necked thermos flask. ***Don't allow it to go through the X-Ray machines at customs. It will destroy its potency.*** When you reach your destination transfer it to a refrigerator as soon as possible. Care should be taken to ensure probiotics are never exposed to temperatures exceeding 80 degrees.

The rest of your supplements can be calculated according to the number of days you intend to be away from home and all placed in one pot, but in separate packs of foil, labeled so you know which is which.

This cuts down on bulk and weight.

Always remember to take some snacks with you and something suitable to drink, you never know if there will be delays.

When traveling to foreign countries, you may have difficulty finding dairy free products such as margarine and soya milk and cheeses. It is advisable to acquire a cold bag, the kind you use to bring frozen foods home from the supermarket in, then you can take a supply of special foods with you.

It is relatively easy to remain on your diet in countries around the Mediterranean such as Spain, Greece, Italy and Israel, because their every day cuisine includes many of the foods approved. In France the chefs are marvelous and willingly cater for your needs, although French bread and cheeses tend to steal your resolve if you are not careful. America could be the worst place for temptation, especially for those with a sweet tooth.

So when planning time away from home, choose your destination carefully. Go only where you can be sure to keep to your diet, then you will really benefit from the trip, coming home feeling well and refreshed.

"Bon Voyage"

KIDS AND CANDIDA

Until recently, Candida and M.E. were thought to be exclusive to adults, but it is becoming increasingly apparent that an ever growing number of children are also sufferers with the conditions often going unrecognized by parents and doctors alike. Usually symptoms are written off as childhood allergies which they will 'grow out of'. They don't grow out of it, the symptoms change, either compounding into other health problems or being suppressed by allopathic medication. Children with recurrent tonsillitis and ear infections are extremely common, but more distressing are the numbers of 3 to 12 year olds with thrush, worm infestation and cystitis. Many are having serious attacks of ulcerative colitis, bleeding from the bowel. All these conditions are Candida related.

Hyperactive children are everywhere in spite of parents being informed of the effects of food additives and colorants. There are so many badly behaved youngsters now, their behaviour is becoming accepted as normal. It is significant that the crime rate among children is higher than ever before.

Also eczema, asthma, hay-fever, bed wetting, acne, dyslexia, inability to concentrate and poor memory have increased. Do these symptoms sound familiar? In an adult we would recognize Candida. Why be surprised that children suffer from it too? You may ask why children should become victims of this relentless parasite, the answer is twenty first century living conditions.

Amalgam fillings in young mouths must take some of the blame. Dentists worldwide are becoming aware of the levels of toxicity caused by mercury poisoning. A colleague of mine Dr. Jack Levenson has spent a lifetime researching the problem and has written an amazing book on the subject. (See the heading - Dental Treatment). It is essential reading for parents who want their children to grow up healthy. Indeed, to preserve their own health also. Mercury is such a toxic substance - should we implant it in our mouth, only inches from the brain? I think not!

In spite of mounting evidence to the contrary, from researchers all over the world, the "old school" of dentists may still argue that amalgam fillings trap the mercury, preventing leakage. Don't believe them. I personally have seen incredible health changes in many adults as a result of the removal of amalgam dental work and I will never again allow it in my mouth. If children haven't yet been subjected to mercury in the mouth don't ever let them be.

Hormone intervention by means of the birth pill and implants must also come under scrutiny. These treatments cause the female body to become deficient in zinc, magnesium and bifido bifodum bacteria, all essential for maintaining a healthy immune system. Women who have taken these forms of contraception will be lacking these nutrients so important to the formation of a healthy foetus. Sensible women cease these forms of contraception for about six months before trying to become pregnant, unfortunately this still does not redress the balance. The deficiencies remain, and a subsequent child is born deficient. *You can only pass on what you yourself have.*

In past generations nature had a way of preventing sickly babies being born by rendering an unhealthy woman unable to conceive. Nowadays thousands of women every year are being given fertility drugs and hormone treatments because they fail to conceive, but the real problem is never addressed. The female reproductive mechanism is failing because of 21st century doctoring methods and living conditions.

Orthodox medicine refuses to take this into account, consequently pregnancies are being achieved by weird and wonderful, unnatural means, in bodies not fit for the task of making a healthy child.

The ultimate result is a generation of children born with deficiencies leading to poor immune responses. Therefore they are condemned to a poor quality of life and health, even before they are born. When they are born, they are subjected to more difficulties because their immune systems are incomplete. Breast milk might take care of it, except, because of hormone treatments, the mother is devoid of bifidus bifodum, so even if she does breast feed, the child doesn't receive it from her.

The child cries continuously because his alimentary tract is not comfortable. It is not being lined with the 'friendly flora' so essential to digestion. The health visitor, if there is one, tells the new mother she doesn't have enough milk and baby is hungry. She advises supplementation with a cow's milk formula. Cows milk is for baby cow's not baby people and the child's system reacts. He throws up, or develops nappy rash, or baby eczema, or excessive mucous, maybe all of them.

Poor child, what an awful start. Soon baby develops a bad behavioural pattern. Crying continuously, rarely sleeping, vomiting possibly at every feed, he may even begin to pass blood in his stools or have diarrhoea or constipation. Along comes our well meaning visitor. Her advice is to regulate the baby's bowel movements with some sugar in his feed.

The yeast parasite (Candida albicans) already present in his gut, loves the sugar and feeds on it, undeterred by the 'friendly flora' which should be present to hold it back. It multiplies and flourishes. Soon the toxins produced by the invader begin to attack the infant's already weak immune system. His body tries to rid itself of the toxic overload. He develops a worse runny nose, a sore throat, an ear infection.

Mother is worried so she takes him to the doctor. He says, "Antibiotics will clear it in a few days." They may do, but in doing so they strip the last vestiges of defence from his immune system.

Then he develops the first in a long line of allergic symptoms. Eczema, asthma, post nasal drip causing perpetual throat clearing and nasal 'snorting,' hyperactivity, phobias about being alone in the dark and behavioural peculiarities that the parents and others are at a loss to know how to deal with. The awful truth is, nobody likes a child like this so he begins to feel unloved. Now he is insecure, he develops a personality problem, so he becomes really naughty to gain attention. His mum can't cope, remember she doesn't feel well herself, she is still deficient.

To keep him quiet she gives him the sweet things he constantly craves, sweets, cakes, biscuits, chocolate etc.. The Candida is multiplying and demanding to be fed. He also becomes hooked on chemically dederived additives. His favourites will be the red and yellow colourants usually found in soft drinks and sweets. The more he has, the worse he becomes and his parents finally seek help. The orthodox medical profession has no answer so they turn to an alternative practitioner like me.

The child's condition may take months to put right and he must be put on a carefully balanced, nutritional programme along with the strict no sugar, no yeast, no cow's milk, diet until his immune system begins to work properly for the first time.

In my experience, children almost always recognize immediately the changes in themselves for the better and are happy to comply. As the aggression diminishes people treat him differently. They don't yell at him all the time and he sometimes gets a hug. He is beginning to feel and be treated like a human being for the first time in his short life.

What about the adults in his life? Some children are surrounded by adults who can't be bothered, or who say, "Oh! The poor little soul, it's not right to deprive him of all the nice things other kids have." They then pop more sugary food into his mouth and say, "Ah! Bless him." I beg you, stop being so sloppy and sentimental. This child is very sick and needs your help. Encourage him to keep the diet so he can have a fair start in life. A start to give him what every human has a God given right to expect, a happy, healthy future.

"Real love gives a child a healthy start"

KINESIOLOGY

This is the name given to the study of locomotion or movement in relation to the structure and working of human muscles. Its root word is from the Greek word 'kinesis' meaning movement. Clearly a subject to interest those with muscular fatigue.

Applied kinesiology is a technique developed in the mid 1960s by Dr. George Goodheart. It incorporates the principles of Chiropractic, Acupuncture, Shiatsu and Massage.

By using this science, a practitioner can achieve helpful results. When muscles are weak, bones can become misaligned, resulting in pressure on the autonomic nervous system and thus causing malfunction of internal organs. This chain reaction causes much more discomfort than is actually attributable to the initial illness. Kinesiology manipulates the muscles into moving the bones back into alignment, thus releasing the nervous system and allowing energy and healing messages from the brain to travel uninterrupted to the organs. This technique has proved very beneficial to clients in the clinic. Massage soothes and comforts, relieving aches and pains. It also helps clear the lymphatic system, speeding up the healing process. I recommend a treatment at least once a month if it is possible in your locality.

At one of Dr. Goodheart's lectures, he repeatedly stressed 'The body cannot lie'. Years in practice have taught me the truth of that statement. Where there is pain or malfunction, there is a cause. Find the cause and put it right and improvement must follow. There is no substitute for the trained hands and knowledge of an experienced practitioner.

Applied Kinesiology is also a means to test foods and other substances for allergic reactions. It can indicate both to the practitioner and the sufferer how much improvement to the immune system has been achieved. This is done by placing the substance either in the mouth or against the skin on a sensitive area of the body, then testing muscles to discern the degree of strength or weakness the substances cause.

Men in particular, are surprised at the extent of the weakness produced when their muscles are tested and the allergens identified by this procedure. They often ask for the test to be repeated claiming they weren't ready for it, but try as they might the result is the same, proving the reliability of the method.

The extent of muscular weakness caused by food allergies can bring the realization that continuous misalignment of bones needing osteopathic treatments can be due to an unrecognized food allergy.

Yes, applied kinesiology is a wonderful science and testifies to the complexity of the human body. It is another way to help you to regain your health.

"The body is intricately simple and simply intricate. If you produce the right measure for the right condition, you get the right response."

(George Goodheart)

" I shall laud you, because in an awesome way, I am wonderfully made. Your works are wonderful as my soul is very well aware."

(King David of Israel..... Psalm 139 v 14)

KNOWLEDGE

People should inform themselves as much as possible about their illness. When you understand the nature of your condition, you know which direction to take in order put your body right. The best way to obtain the knowledge you need is to read up on it.

How do you know which books to choose. Conflicting information can be very confusing. The books I have found most helpful are these:-

"The Yeast Syndrome" by John Parks Trowbridge & Morton Walker published by Bantam.
"Candida albicans, Yeast and Your health," by Gill Jacobs published by Optima.
"Candida albicans, Could Yeast be your Problem?" by Leon Chaitow published by Thorsons.
"Maximum Immunity" by Michael A. Weiner, Ph. D. published by Gateway.

There is danger in reading too much, because so many different treatments may be suggested. If you try and fail to achieve results with several, you could become disheartened and give up, or you may spend money on supplements that prove either, not potent enough to do the job, or unnecessary.

It is also important to gain knowledge about your own body, its needs and reactions. Try to train yourself, if you have not already done so, to be aware of changes both from within yourself and in your environment. For instance, sleepiness and muscular weakness can be the first symptoms of allergy. When you eat something or come into contact with a substance you react to, you will be aware of the cause and avoid it in future. This will save you long periods of debility. It has often been said, "A little knowledge is a dangerous thing," I don't agree...

"Accurate knowledge can lead you back to good health"

LETTERS

During the years I have been in practice, it has been my privilege to help a great number of people back to good health. Many of them have written to me and I have treasured those letters because, not only have they been an encouragement to me to continue my work, but they are proof that the methods I have adopted really do work. I have included some of them here so that you too may find encouragement from them.

Many describe symptoms that you will be able to identify with. Also the frustrations experienced whilst awaiting results. Above all else, I hope you will be reassured by them knowing improvement is possible and a normal life can be regained.

*"They found the way back to good health
and so can you"*

The text and grammar of these letters has been left unchanged.
They are reproduced as they were written.

Mrs P.G.
Canvey Island

Dear Mrs Hampton,

I want to thank you so much for helping my daughter Cheryl to regain her health.

As you know she had suffered from Psoriasis for many years and by the time we came to you she was covered except the lower half of her face. None of the steroids and tar preparations had ever helped. But within four weeks of visiting you her skin and scalp were completely clear and have remained so ever since.

The flakiness started to go as soon as Cheryl took the multi-vitamins and zinc, but the patches disappeared completely when she cut out the foods you discovered she was sensitive to.

Now without using any creams or medicines she is clear of the ailment that I was told she would suffer from for the rest of her life.

There are no words to express my gratitude, maybe Cheryl can say it better herself:-

Thank you for making my skin like everyone elses. Now I can wear my swimsuit next summer and won't have to keep myself all covered up.

Thank you very much.

Lot's of love

Cheryl

I'm looking forward so much to showing you the living evidence when I bring Cheryl to see you in December.

Our Sincerest gratitude

Mrs L.H.
Crawley

Dear Mrs Hampton,

I thought I must write to thank you for all you have done for me so far, and how well I look and feel.

As you remember when I first came to you I was a sorry sight:- eyes red and blood-shot, severe constipation and constant tiredness, always sleeping during the day - and belts of depression. In fact I really don't know how I got through each day.

Now all that has gone, my eyes are bright with a twinkle, skin glows, constipation improved and most of all I have energy, something I have not had since I was a child. I am now on the go all day and only sleep at night.

My marriage has improved and I have more time for my family.

When you consider that my family doctor said I had a 'delicate constitution' and gave me stronger laxative, I began to despair.

Thank you Jo for what you have achieved in so few months, I had no idea one could feel so good

Yours sincerely

Linda

Dereham, Norfolk, England.
2.March 2001

Dear Jo,
Just over two years ago, when I was 34, I began to feel very unwell. Everything I ate gave me indigestion and wind. I was depressed and tired, with no energy to enjoy socializing, which made me feel ill afterwards if eating and drinking were involved. I often had 'flu like symptoms, feeling shivery and sick. I gradually became worse, needing to go to bed in the afternoons, and going to bed at 6pm, only to wake next morning feeling I wanted to stay in bed a all day. I also had an itchy, sore rash on the palms of my hands, and continually suffered mouth ulcers.

I saw my doctor, who first diagnosed an ulcer, then gall stones and gave me numerous tests and drugs, before telling me it was all in my mind and that I was obviously depressed!

A friend suggested I should go and see Jo hampton, who after carefully discovering what all my symptoms were, diagnosed a Candida problem, which had caused food allergies, and suggested I followed an anti Candida diet, coupled with taking special natural medicines.

It was a long process before I began feeling well again, and sometimes I nearly gave up hope. I would say that I felt worse at some points in the beginning of the treatment, but I am so glad I stuck with the diet and did not give up hope that I would be well in the end. Jo was very supportive and helpful and Vega tests showed that my immune system was slowly recovering, even though I still sometimes felt quite poorly.

Now 21 months after I first began, I have finally rid myself of all my food allergies and the Candida albicans. I am feeling fit and well, and am able to enjoy going out for meals and going on holiday again. I have loads of energy and feel happy again, which is vital for a mother of three young children!

I am so glad I went to see jo, even though I hardly had the strength to carry out her intructions. It was really hard, but I knew I could not carry on feeling as awful as I did before my treatment.

Best Wishes

Marigold

TO JO AND GOOD HEALTH

I used to be deathly and needed a vet
Listen, you aint heard nothing yet
I was a wreck and no mistake
One more minute and I was ready to break
Just one look and you could see I was a
gonner
being prepared wholesale for animal fodder
Yes, a walking medical sad mystery
"He's neurotic, nothings wrong!" Said my GP

And yet there was hope yes, yes surely!
Just down the motorway with Jo. In Crawley.
I came, I saw, Jo gave hope and all those pills!
I'm a new man folks. With disappearing ills!!!!

Now listen, patients all, you've heard my tale,
I'm better, living, and no longer pale!
She's a great gal, a goldmine tis true -
All who enter don't doubt - I hope that's not
you!!!
She'll cure what you've got and much, much
more,
But boy, there's no one better to make you sore

Bless your little cotton socks!

A thousand thanks, from a getting well, grate-
ful disciple,
(and his grateful wife)

Alan + Partner

Susan D
Basildon

Dear Jo,

Had to write to say, how much better I am
feeling, and only after 6 months of
treatment. I am very glad that you have
taken the time and effort. I was really fed
up with orthodox treatment.

Now, after visiting you and having your
treatment, I now know what is wrong with
me and how to cure it. (Candida).

Here I am, I can see the light at the end
of the tunnel of illness, and it is refreshing
to me.

Carry on the good work.

Yours faithfully,

Susan D

105

Isleworth
Middlesex

Dear Jo,

Just a few lines to say thanks for all of your help and encouragement and your wonderful treatment. It really worked!

I have been transformed from a person who had no energy, had asthma, many food-allergies and allergies to dogs, cats, dust etc., in just over three months, to a person who radiates good health.

I haven't used my inhaler now for over two months which is unbelievable, I used to use it up to five times a day before. I have bags of energy and I can go near any dog or cat and suffer no ill-effects.

My skin is much better, no more blemishes/dark bags under my eyes and I can now wear any earrings I like, (I haven't been able to wear any for over a year as my ears used to weep and swell up even with gold earrings) and for any lady who is reading this, my PMT is almost non-existant - no more asthma for 2 weeks non-stop before my period.

I hope my letter will encourage anyone suffering with asthma allergies etc. to take the plunge and try your wonderful treatment, because it really works.

Thank you and good luck to you and your future patients.

Miss Sue A

These two poems were written by a ten year old girl, "Fear" before, & "Courage", after treatment

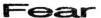
Fear
March 1989

Breath taken away
I feel Shaken up
Strength Disappearing
Mind blank.
My body feels like it's empty
Fingers cold like stone
I feel like someone has taken
my courage away
Nerve wrecking
I'm bubbling with FEAR

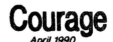
Courage
April 1990

I feel strong
I could run a race
My mind is full of ideas
I feel hot like a fire
As I play in the garden
It's nice with courage
It's lovely

South Benfleet

Dear Jo,

Please find enclosed case history of how we managed to get our Isaac.

I hope it helps to prove your point, and finally be taken seriously by the medical profession.

At the age of eighteen I was prescribed the pill. On occasion I suffered extremely painful periods, and the pill seemed the only answer. However, after four years I was married and we both decided we would like to start a family as soon as possible.

In our first year of marriage, my husband Steve became extremely ill. He had been diagnosed as having colitis two years previously and had been receiving treatment accordingly. This treatment consisted of a course of hormone tablets, salzapyrine which, according to the specialist, he would have to take for the rest of his life. However, his health slowly deteriorated almost to the point of him being admitted for an operation. His weight had gone from 11 1/2 stone to 8 1/2 stone in only about 2 weeks.

There was hope, given to us by a family friend who recommended we see a homeopath. That was when we met you and you diagnosed Steve as having Candida. You were very helpful and after the special diet and a course of homeopathic medicines he was back to his normal self. He was much healthier and more aware of his own diet, and if ever his symptoms return now, he knows how to cure himself. It was by coincidence at this time that I overheard a talk show on the radio where the guest speaker was a doctor. Someone called asking about 'Salzapyrine' and questioning whether it was true that this course of treatment could make you sterile. The answer from the radio doctor was 'yes salzapyrine can effect fertility'. On hearing this, my husband brought the subject up at his next appointment with the specialist. Yes they can affect fertility, was the reply from the consultant. So why were they prescribed to a newly-married man in his twenties? It was standard procedure, everyone, regardless of circumstance, was given this treatment unless they asked or inquired about an alternative. With that, my husband ceased his treatment with the NHS.

Within months of Steve stopping his hormone treatment I fell pregnant. We were overjoyed. After two years of trying for a baby, with no luck, we were on the verge of going to a fertility clinic. But we just put our bad luck down to the fact of Steve's illness and the hormone treatment he had been receiving.

At ten weeks gestation I began to bleed, it was diagnosed as a threatened miscarriage. The only treatment for which was bed rest. This I did, but two weeks later I did miscarry and was taken into hospital for a D & C.

The baby, they told me, was perfectly formed to about six to eight weeks gestation, it had died some weeks before I actually lost it. There was no explanation as to why this happened, only that it was quite common to miscarry, it was 'just one of those things'.

I found it hard to come to terms with the loss. The only way to overcome this was to have a baby. So we tried again as soon as possible.

⟶

107

After a year and a half of trying, and doctor saying there was no physical reason why I should not be able to fall pregnant, I fell pregnant eventually and determined that I would not lose this one, I took things very easy for the first few weeks. This had no effect, however, I miscarried for the second time, under the same circumstances as the first. At this point I began to lose hope of ever being able to carry. The doctor in the hospital told me it wasn't unusual to miscarry twice, and that they wouldn't be able to do any investigations until I had lost a third baby.

What was I to do? I wanted a baby so much I couldn't face going through the physical and emotional turmoil of miscarriage again. My GP, I would like to add, was very supportive and did everything she could to push investigations forward. These investigations only went as far as me having a smear test and my husband having a sperm-count. Nothing unusual was found with the results of either. Just continue with the temperature charts I was told.

I knew I was able to get pregnant, the only problem was keeping up the pregnancy. I was left no choice but to help myself with my problem, and so I decided to seek homeopathic advice.

I made an appointment to see you and you gave me a simple allergy test and found, like my husband, I had a yeast allergy. Although my symptoms were not as severe as my husbands.

You advised me on my diet, which consisted of basically telling me what foods I should avoid, and a course of supplements.

★ Within a month my period came, and before my follow-up check-up with you I had fallen pregnant again. I couldn't believe it, I fell so quickly! The next problem was to keep my pregnancy going. I took your advice and stuck to the diet until the danger period was over. Those first weeks seemed to last forever. I worried over every slightest thing. The moment of truth arrived when I went for my first scan at 10 weeks. He wasn't very big, but there, for all to see was a tiny heartbeat.

I was told everything seemed normal, but I was to continue having regular scans just to make sure.

There was no need to worry. The pregnancy continued without a hitch. On the 25th of February 1991, 10 days late, Isaac was born. Two years almost to the day from when my first baby was due. Labour lasted five hours. I needed no drugs and Isaac weighed a healthy 7 lb 12 ozs.

I'm convinced that if I hadn't gone to you for help, we would still be just a couple and not the family we are today.

My Candida symptoms would probably have escalated making conceiving even more difficult. Or worse, I may have carried a child, again which may have been too weak to survive.

Good Luck

Sue B

108

Crawley Down,
West Sussex.

Dear Mrs Hampton,

I felt I must write to say how thrilled we are with progress our daughter, Sally, has made since we first came to you two months ago.

For the first time in five years her skin allergy has completely cleared up, and even her pigment has started to return (which the doctors said never would!)

After years of going to and fro to hospital, and having endless tubes of cortisone cream, your approach - to get to and remove the cause - makes so much sense.

I must admit that my husband had heard of your treatment and philosophy, but now he's so thankful that Sally doesn't have to face her teenage years with the embarrassment of rashes and large white patches.

I will gladly recommend you to any of my friends. Keep up the good work!

Yours sincerely

Mrs. Pat G.

Dear Jo,

I thought it was about time I wrote and thanked you for all your help. I feel like a different person and it's all thanks to you.

I remember so well that wet and dreary day I drove up to see you last January. I felt so ill I really don't know how I made it. You were so kind and understanding, I at last felt I had found someone who knew what was wrong and who would be able to help. The next few months were bad as I kept to your candida treatment regime, but after that, things quickly picked up and now I'm a new person.

Thank you very much,
Lesley,
London.

Newbury,
London.

Dear Jo Hampton,

I wanted to write to thank you for the excellent treatment, guidance and support you have provided for me over the past months.

When I first attended your clinic in September '87, I was feeling absolutely dreadful. I was highly stressed, emotionally drained, suffering from severe bouts of depression and experiencing a level of confusion and unhappiness I had not previously known.

My physical health was very poor. Sore throats, severe thrush, skin rash and exhaustion. I was hardly able to get through each day - needing to sleep a minimum of 10 hours each night and requiring stretches of 12-15 hours sleep at weekends.

I started your candida diet and the full treatment of Capricin, Bifido, garlic and vitamins. Within the first three months I had drastically improved but was still "not right". It has been a long, slow and difficult process but over the months, I have improved to the point that by February '88 I felt 90% better. The candida had receded, I lost weight and my skin had cleared.

Over the past twelve months, I have had my "ups and downs", but when I stick to a sensible diet and continue with the supplements you recommend, I feel better.

Recently I have had an attack of vaginal thrush due to inadvisably taking Royal Jelly. I have felt slightly under the weather, but my immune system is now strong enough to fight the condition without the dreadful side-effects of the past.

I am taking Capricin for a month as an extra precaution.

I know without any doubt that my recovery is due to your diagnosis and treatment.

My doctor still refuses to believe in my condition. An appalling response as I visited my doctor many, many times while feeling so ill, yet she was unable to help at all. In fact she made things worse by constantly prescribing antibiotics.

I also want to praise your personal approach to myself and your patients. Your constant enthusiasm, support and positivity has been invaluable - especially at the times when I felt really low and like giving up.

Whenever I telephoned you, you would always give a helpful, positive response and provide the much-needed guidance, support and encouragement.

I have recommended your treatment to anyone I know who thinks they are suffering from Candida.

Keep up your wonderful work.

With best wishes,

Lynn S.

Ifield,
Crawley,
West Sussex.

Dear Mrs Hampton,

I thought I would write to thank you for the great improvement in my general health since I started your anti-candida-albicans diet.

When I came to see you initially I had been seeking alternative treatment for the sinus problems I had suffered for nearly two years. I had seen an ENT specialist and an allergy specialist, but they could not agree on the cause or suggest a permanent solution. Through my GP I received medication for the rhinitis and although he was helpful and sympathetic, felt he could do no more for me. It was my cat's vet who recommended you to me. He had rhinitis and had seen exactly the same specialists as me, with the same lack of results. He was well enough after your treatment to recommend the diet.

I was very surprised when you suggested during our first meeting that not only the rhinitis, but all the other minor health problems I had were part of the same syndrome, namely Candida Albicans. I was delighted that having sought help for the sinus problems you were also confident you could clear up the other ailments I had, which individually didn't seem sufficiently bad to worry my overworked GP about, but which collectively were getting me down. I had put many of my problems down to galloping middle-age.

Within days of starting your treatment, I felt an improvement in my general well-being; I felt that my brain had been switched on again after months of mental confusion; my concentration improved; my eyesight improved; I lost the feeling of nervous anxiety which had been my companion for many months and felt more calm and composed. As the days went by my sleep pattern improved and for the first time in months, was sleeping right through the night. I felt younger and as if a great weight had been lifted from my shoulders. General aches and pains disappeared. I became more aware of myself and my surroundings; I became more interested in myself, my home and my life generally. My co-ordination and memory

———————————➤

improved. My mouth and throat, which had for months been so dry that at times it was almost impossible to carry on a conversation of any length, improved and the hoarseness in my voice disappeared completely. My nose is slowly improving, having been waterlogged for over eighteen months it's quite a relief.

I had for some years found overhead light, both indoors and outdoors, very uncomfortable but find now that this doesn't bother me so much. I have noticed that when I'm working in the garden I don't wear my sun hat or sun-glasses quite so often and I'm sure that's not entirely due to the awful weather we've had this autumn!

A very welcome and unexpected bonus of the treatment is that my periods have changed from a seven day drag to a four day event I hardly notice. I had previously suffered almost fourteen days of PMT symptoms, including sore breasts, bloating with weight gain of about five pounds, increasing bad temper and irritability. My dear long-suffering husband, recognising the signs would keep a very low profile. I tried to arrange my life so that I didn't have to cope with the stress of visitors or entertaining around the time of my period. My last two periods have arrived on their due day, without any PMT warning.

I've lost about eight pounds in weight, although I didn't anticipate this, even though I'm eating much more. In recent months I'd been slowly gaining weight and for the first time in my life had to watch my calorie intake. I love cooking and eating (vegetarian) so my recently revived metabolism is extremely useful.

The greatest improvement of all is in my energy level. I have been tired for as long as I can remember, but have been able to overcome it. However, during the last year or so I have been persistently exhausted. It became increasingly difficult to cope with my daily domestic routine and I had no energy for pastimes of gardening and sewing. I had reached the point where, although I tried to plan my days as best I could, more often than not found I was just too tired to cope or too confused to remember the days plan. It was taking me ages to complete even simple jobs like washing up after breakfast. Cleaning the house became a major event of outstanding proportions. Soon after starting your diet my energy level

---

increased substantially and now after three months of treatment I feel so full of energy there are days when I don't know how to use it all!! I constantly amaze myself with the amount of work I am now able to get through and still feel ready for more. I have stopped yawning. Until I started your diet my life had become one long yawn.

Over the Christmas period we have seen family and friends and every one has said how much better I'm looking. (one relative remarked that I have stopped yawning). I've even had friends on the telephone say to me "You are sounding very perky these days".

My husband is a great admirer of your treatment and openly tells family and friends how quickly the improvement in my well-being showed after starting the diet. I don't think I've ever felt so strong or so well in my entire life. In three months you have transformed my health and vitality and you will never know how grateful I am to you.

All this good health by natural means; a few changes in the diet; no drugs, no side effects. It almost seems too good to be true.

I can't begin to thank you enough for the great improvement you have made in my health and wellbeing.

Looking forward to seeing you again soon and in the meantime take this opportunity of wishing you the happiest and healthiest New Year.

Yours sincerely,

Mo

1

Crowborough,
Sussex.

Dear Jo,

I thought it was time I put pen to paper and wrote about my experiences coping with candida, so that it may reassure and influence those who may be suffering or possibly going through the healing stages.

Firstly, I would like to thank you Jo for your wonderful support, you have given to both myself and my mother, through these troubled times. You have been fantastic, as well as so sensitive to our needs and concerns. We are now enjoying our new lease of life and feeling cleansed and refreshed.

My mother has suffered from the most horrendous and crippling migraines for many years, and thanks to you, she is now a different woman she is radiant with health and vitality, as well as migraine free.

2

I will briefly outline my past since birth, as I feel this is all relevant.

I was born in 1968, with club feet. I was operated on as a baby until the age of twenty. My operations have been a great success.

My problems occurred when I was sixteen when I experienced a nasty case of acne. Following doses of antibiotics and cortisone creams, my face then blew up like a panda and the symptoms got worse. It appeared that cutting out sugary and fatty food cleared it up.

Since then I have been particularly cautious of my diet. It was a year later that I had my first attack of candida. Having drunk a glass of wine, I felt a deep cramp feeling in my stomach, that then worked up my chest into my shoulders and arms. The pain was awful, as too was the dizziness and fever that accompanied it.

Over the years I have become aware of how to handle the attacks. But on my

3

return from America, where I had so many, and I was being constantly ill with colds and sickness, I then got an appointment with you.

I was becoming more miserable, as spots around my mouth flared up and down all depending on what I had eaten. I was distressed and felt out of control of my life.

Other reactions I experienced, were hyperactivity, lethargy, lack of concentration and poor memory.

It was May 1991 when I first visited you. You put me on the special candida diet as well as the essential vitamins. I felt great, and then the withdrawal symptoms set in. I had a headache and felt generally under the weather. Two weeks into the diet, I then started experiencing the toxin release. I was unaware of how they came out, that is until they appeared as water blisters on my face. Shocked as I was, more came, burst and then formed thick crusty scabs, as large as 50p coins.

4

Seeing this horrified myself and family but after a month it had cleared and you assured me that it would not scar, which thankfully it has not.

It is now November, and I am feeling really well. I have not had any attacks and am now eating far healthier than I have done in years.

Today, I am still on the diet and supplements, and will continue to take them until my bodies immune system is built up.

Anyway, all my many, many thanks go out to you and your husband Ben, who have been so kind and supportive throughout my illness.

Thank you, Thank you.

With all my fondest of love,

Rebecca
XXX

Kenley,
Surrey.

Dear Jo,

Just a few lines to say thank-you for all the help and support you and your team gave me to make me well again. You were always a great help to me and when things were tough you always helped me through. For anyone who is considering the ... regime, I'd just like to say that in my case the first few days were awful, then I began to feel really well, all my worst symptoms seemed to clear very quickly, headaches, nausea, lethargy, sinus problems etc and generally I felt really well. I expected this to continue, but I found after a couple of months that although no actual symptoms returned, I felt at times more tired and listless than I had ever felt before. I knew that this was the candida dying off, but at times I thought why am I doing this? I knew I was sticking to the diet rigidly and taking all the supplements as directed, but at times I felt really discouraged. The most encouraging signs came after a few months when my food allergies began to clear, this encouraged me on to continue the treatment.

Shortly after this I began to have more energy and enthusiasm for things, I started to look better and people began saying I looked better than they had seen me for a long time. This progress continued and although I am still very careful what I eat, the candida is now under control and everything about me is 100% better than I can ever remember it being before.

The treatment is not an easy thing to go through, but the end results are well worth it.

Thank you all again,

Wendy

★ M.E. complicated by Candida and Allergies

115

Crawley
Sussex

Dear Mrs Hampton,

I wish to thank you from the bottom of my heart for making me feel so well in such a short time.

I had suffered for years with a string of ailments and doctors and specialists could not help me. No-one understood how I felt, not even my husband and we are very close, except of course yourself. I felt really old and had given up ever finding a cure and my life was just a drudge. But you have changed all that, it was as though you could see inside me and knew my body better than I did. I would never have dreamed that all my problems were caused by my own hand, the food that I ate plus drugs etc. I dreaded the thought of giving up certain foods but I was willing to try anything after all I had nothing to lose, except that I lost I stone of unwanted fat. So yes, I had to give myself a talking to and pull my belt in, but I couldn't have done it without you. I cannot speak or write too highly of your treatment. I am extremely pleased with the results even though the treatment hasn't finished yet.

So thanks to you I can look forward to a new and healthier future and I'm so glad to have found you.

I look forward to my next visit. Many, many thanks.

Mrs Jean S.

Crawley.
Sussex.

Dear Jo,

I thought that I must write to you to thank you for helping me to recover from the "Candida" albicans" complaint. It is so nice to get through the day without feeling sick and giddy. I also felt that I had permanent flu. I ached and had no energy.

Also my sinuses were permanently blocked and I suffered chronic sinusitis.

I now find I have more energy and don't feel so tired, and I don't catch every cold or virus there is going.

It is so nice to feel well at long last. I never thought I could feel like this.

Jo I can never thank you enough.

Much love,

Jane

XX

Mrs Carol L.,
Canvey,
Essex.

Dear Jo,

I would just like to thank you for all your help and kindness I've received during my treatment, because I'm so well now and it's made me realise Jo how ill I was.

Because I was house-bound and not able to live a normal life, I was so weak physically. I could not walk, but now I feel my strength coming back. I've not felt as good as this in years.

But I must admit Jo there were times when I thought I was not going to recover because the first three months I felt terrible, but there were some good days, but with your encouragement and also my husband, and many friends who also receive your treatment, I could see how well they had recovered. I was determined to get well too, and prepared to do anything, and I followed thy diet and supplements to thy letter, and any good advice from you to make my life a healthy one.

So once again Jo, thank you.

Warm love from Carol L.

LIFESTYLE

O.K! So you want to enjoy life! To do it you have to be well. You need to assess the way your chosen lifestyle is affecting your health. Ask yourself why you have become ill. Is it due to the way you have been living?

Have you smoked heavily or drunk alcohol excessively over a long period of time? Do you crawl into bed in the early hours. Have you been working extended hours or traveling long distances to and from work adding extra hours to your working day? Is your private life a complicated muddle, or your love life perpetually causing you stress? All these could be contributing to the loss of vital energy that has led to your present poor health.

There are some factors in all our lives over which we have little control. Things like caring for elderly parents, raising difficult children, mortgage rates etc... But many of the stresses we live with, we bring on ourselves and if we want good health we must be prepared to make changes.

First assess the sum total of your way of life, and its affect, then do something constructive about reducing the stress load. If you smoke, choose to stop. The same goes for drinking to excess. Go to bed at a reasonable hour. Refuse some overtime or delegate responsibility at work. Possibly find a job nearer home, or move closer to work. With time and thought, sort out your home muddle and stabilize your love life.

Find a few non smoking, moderate drinking, less demanding, non-party going friends. As much fun, or more, can be had by sharing a healthy evening meal or an exchange of ideas and news with a few well chosen friends at home. You may think this advice old fashioned, but years ago, Candida, M.E. and allergies were not at epidemic proportions. Maybe it was because people led more tranquil lives. You can't enjoy anything while you are ill, so....

"Change your habits for a better quality of life"

LYMPHATIC DRAINAGE

This is an important part of your plan to regain good health. Your lymphatic system is an intricate filter mechanism made up of tiny vessels circulating milky fluid throughout the body. This fluid helps maintain the correct balance in tissues to defend against disease, but also carries away waste products and harmful bacteria.

When a person suffers from an immuno deficiency condition the lymphatic system can become overloaded with waste, clogging up and preventing proper drainage. This often happens when sufferers choose to treat themselves without benefit of a practitioner who incorporates massage.

The person reaches a stage where no further progress can be made. When attention is given to lymphatic drainage, then improvement begins again.

The massage technique used is often painful the first time it is performed. It should be. A quick rub down by a local beautician or a gentle aromatherapist will not suffice. Few practitioners know how, or have the strength to perform this treatment well. Don't pay for a substitute which does no good.

Another method of stimulating lymphatic drainage is to acquire a 'rebounder'. These are like mini trampolines, you simply step on and bounce up and down for a few minutes each day. The action of defying gravity not only improves your heart rate, and gets lymphatic fluid moving, but it also tones up slack muscles.

"There's no gain without pain"

MAKE-UP AND MORALE

When I was a child I can remember my mother owning a recording by the music hall artist Stanley Holloway. It was a comic song called "My Word You Do Look Queer." You may have heard it too. The lyric tells of a man whose friends keep telling him how ill he looks, until one comes along and says how well he looks. The very last line of the song is a jubilant shout of, *"My word I do feel well."*

Much comedy is based on observation of truth. That old song is an example. When you look dreary and down people feel sorry for you, but they also say negative things, tending to drag you still further down.

You need them to tell you how much better you look than when they saw you last. Up building comments to leave you encouraged and feeling positive. For this to happen, you have to present as cheerful a face as possible.

For a man it means washing, shaving, combing his hair and putting on a clean shirt. A woman needs to make a small effort with her hair and put on a little lip-stick and perhaps eye make-up. I know it's a chore when you feel low, but a positive attitude on your part can have really good results on your health.

If you look cheerful and bright, maybe a whole day will pass without anyone mentioning your health and for a while you too may be able to forget it and feel as bright as you look.

This must create a more positive atmosphere around you which will be of untold benefit to your health. So be like Elena Rigby of Beatles fame. Keep your face in a jar behind the door and don't let anyone in until you have it firmly in place.

If you look good, you'll feel great"

MASSAGE

Massage is marvelous! Of all the therapies I have learned and mentioned in this book, massage is dearest to my heart. It can achieve so much. Valuable for people of all ages, with all manner of illnesses, but never more beneficial than for those with M.E. and Candida. Massage can relieve the awful aching, tiredness and heavy feelings they experience. It lowers blood pressure, reduces stress, relaxes or stimulates, frees mental tension and promotes feelings of well-being. It is also instrumental in the disposal of waste matter accumulated in the lymphatic system.

All this is so important, but best of all, massage gives comfort. When you are being massaged you are in no doubt that someone else cares.

In India it is part of the ancient healing art of Ayah Veda. The Japanese incorporate it as part of the practice of Shiatsu. Swedish massage is known and valued all over the western world. In China, those born blind are trained in it, because as trained masseurs they can then become valuable members of the community although disabled.

The practice of massaging with the essential oils of plants to bring beneficial changes to clients has recently been revived on a large scale under the name of Aromatherapy. Many think this to be a new form of therapy, but the Romans were well known for using massage at their public baths. And even further back, around 480 B.C. the Bible records massage being used on the future Queen Esther, the Jewish consort of King Ahasuerus of the Medo-Persian empire.

Massage is one of the oldest of all medical practices, and is known to all of us from a very early age. Many of us remember our mother smoothing our hair from our forehead, with a gentle touch when we suffered childhood illnesses, or the comfort of being lulled to sleep by a loving hand moving back and forth soothingly.

It is now a scientifically established fact, babies who are hugged, touched and massaged by their parents do better and grow up healthier than those who are not. Not only do children thrive on being touched, but elderly people flourish on it too. Try hugging, or holding an elderly relative's hand and you will find out how important human contact is to us all. They will cling to your touch, often reluctant to let go, their need is so great.

You may recall childhood accidents. Perhaps you bumped your head, or skinned your knee. Your mother's first aid treatment was often simply to 'rub it better'. Soon you were running back to your games with no pain, secure in the knowledge that somebody cared.

Massage can be viewed, not only as an essential part of restorative treatment when you are ill, but as maintenance to guard against the stresses and strains of 21st century living.

Those who attend the clinic benefit from a massage technique incorporating lymphatic drainage, acupressure, reflexology and relaxation. Their recovery is speeded up by approximately one third.

Many times, even when people have totally recovered from their original illnesses, they continue to have regular massage, because they have come to recognize the benefits.

Never underestimate the value of good massage. It is a means of prevention as well as a cure.

"Massage is a 'stroke' of genius"

M.E. - WHAT IS IT?

This is a question I am asked repeatedly. I sometimes answer *Misery Epitomized.* Those who suffer from it agree.

In medical terms the initials M.E. Are short for Myalgic Encephalomyelitis. Myalgic means muscular pain and Encephalomyelitis means inflammation of the brain and spinal cord. The muscular pain is a direct result of spinal inflammation, but what causes the inflammation in the first place? There are various causes which I will deal with later.

The initial onset of the condition is, according to my clinical records, precipitated by what is usually diagnosed as being 'flu', a virus or an attack of glandular fever. None of these diagnosis proves comprehensively accurate as the sufferer soon becomes aware when his health progressively deteriorates.

Spinal inflammation causes interference to the delicate mechanism of the autonomic nervous system, the means by which the brain sends messages governing every bodily function and regulates organs. This explains why the whole body becomes affected and why the symptoms are so varied.

Now back to the cause, or causes of the inflammation. I do not believe there is only one cause. The general symptoms are similar in all sufferers but the cause differs from person to person.

For one person it could be caused by over exposure to environmental electromagnetism, for another, organophosphates, yet another may have been affected by immunization as in the case of the Gulf War victims. Some will be reacting to mercury toxicity from leaking amalgam dental fillings, and others from mixed metals causing a 'battery' to form in the mouth putting a block on the brain activity. (See heading Electromagnetism.)

I believe M.E to be a collective title given to all of these modern practices that create interference in the human immune system. The common denominator is the suppression of the immune system but

123

each person must have the original cause identified and then be treated accordingly.

This weakening of the human immune system is peculiar to our age for a number of reasons. One is, we are the third or fourth generation (depending on our age) who have been subjected to the use of synthetic drugs. The most insidious of these has been antibiotics. Those initially treated with them survived their illnesses but their immunity was weakened. The weakness has been passed on through the generations with a cumulative effect. Each generation adding their own quota of drugs to the overall load, until we have a generation born with the weakest immune responses ever.

The same argument may be true of blood transfusions too. It has been proved that Jehovah's Witnesses who refuse blood during major surgery, recover much faster than those who accept a transfusion. The recovery rate is directly linked to the 'foreign' blood having a suppressing effect on immunity. Could it be, this is another source of congenital immune breakdown? Could this also be why T cells become confused and give wrong orders to B cell defenders. (See heading Immune System.)

Also to be taken into account must be the heavy load of global pollution which is depressing the health and immunity of every individual on the planet. Mans interference in the food chain with the use of additives and factory farming is adding more overwhelming burdens. It only takes the minimum of extra stress on a weak immune system and the whole careful balance collapses.

The primary group diagnosed with M.E. are young, active people with high powered lifestyles. Stress, research has established, coupled with emotional turbulence, can contribute to chemical changes in the brain. Hence the encephalomyelitis.

Many protest they are not exposed to stress, but the world is full of it. Who can escape it? Much of our life is spent in a stressful state. Just half an hour on a motor-way can cause stress and blood pressure levels to rise to astronomical heights. Take a look at the average persons love life and you will conclude emotional upsets must be part of the equation.

Throughout the civilized world, marriages have never before been so unstable. Work pressure is greater than ever before because of job shortages. People who have to work, continuously overtax themselves to prove their worth, constantly aware others are waiting to fill their place. The adrenal glands, thyroid and thymus, all vital to immune system function, are put under incredible stress. No wonder the human body suddenly decides it needs a long rest.

You may now appreciate why drugs do not improve the situation. They only contribute to it. Now, you may also understand why so many M.E. sufferers have a Candida problem.

With immunity in such a depressed state, it is the ideal time for the opportunist fungus to make its move. Invasion is easy. Defences are down and overgrowth can flourish in a very short time. In a laboratory it can grow from a single cell to a kilo in weight overnight. *If it can happen so fast in a laboratory, how much faster can it happen in its natural habitat?*

Whether or not M.E. is complicated by Candida it is still of paramount importance to strengthen and restore the immune system. This means the diet and supplements recommended in this book are a very necessary part of recovery, but there will be variations added when the cause of your condition has been determined and the site of breakdown is identified.

To this end, you must find a practitioner who is knowledgeable and skilled in the diagnosis and treatment of M.E.

"It is working for others, it will work for you"

MENOPAUSE - The Candida Connection

Women attending the clinic repeatedly ask questions about the 'bad time' so many of them experience during the change of life.

To answer the question it would be good to ask other questions. For instance, have women always suffered as much during that time of their lives? Or is it another consequence of modern living?

Although the middle years have always been difficult for women, I do not think they have ever been as traumatic as they have become today.

Let's look at the average life of a woman in the changing years. She was born to a more frugal diet than is common today. If she suffered from ear or throat infections in childhood, antibiotics would have been administered with their devastating effects on 'friendly flora'. This went unnoticed, although when Fleming first advocated the use of penicillin he also recommended that live yoghurt be eaten to replace the lost bacterium. Very few people were made aware of this recommendation, live yoghurt was not as popular or available as it is now. So this young girl entered puberty with an imbalance of bacterium, leaving her susceptible to yeast overgrowth.

She may have been one of the first generation of young women to have access to birth control by means of 'the pill'. This made sexual activity possible without fear of pregnancy. A new promiscuous society was born. Even if she didn't use it for contraceptive reasons, it may have been prescribed to regulate her menstrual cycle. Although acclaimed as 'safe', many women will testify to the horrendous side effects artificial hormones caused.

Thrush became a major recurrent problem. Headaches and migraine, weight changes, P.M.S., endometriosis, thrombosis. Many of these symptoms indicated that candidiasis was present, although it was not until 1983 that serious research was done and the extent of the problem began to emerge. It was then, the problem became known as Candida albicans and was attributed in part to the use of hormones and antibiotics.

After looking at her health history let's turn to her lifestyle. Not only does she marry and have a family, but she holds down a full time job too. She is liberated with new rights and financial independence, but also new responsibilities, causes of stress never before experienced by women. She is expected to keep her job outside the home until she is sixty. No chance to put her feet up in the afternoon like her grandmother did when she had an 'off day'.

She is also pressured by a youth orientated society to behave and look like a teenager or her husband will trade her in for a 'new model', or perhaps he already has, causing her terrible trauma. These are only some of the problems facing middle aged women today.

The job may entail several hours a day driving, or sitting in a smoke filled office in front of a computer giving off 'electric smog'. She may be required to deal with complaining, rude members of the public, standing on her feet all day in a shop, or doing repetitive, boring things in a factory whilst being exposed to chemicals.

If she is lucky, she may enjoy her job, but she still has to go home to cope with argumentative teenagers, ailing elderly relatives, cooking a meal and cleaning the house.

Finally she collapses into bed, but she is unable to sleep because she is over stressed and can't 'switch off'. When she does manage to sleep she is awakened by a hot flush and has to get out and change either her nightdress or the bedclothes or both. Then it's morning and the whole process begins again. Is it any wonder her body protests?

Modern woman is stress plagued, and stress is another contributing factor in Candida overgrowth.

Lastly we should examine her diet. Because she is so busy she relies on prepackaged, frozen, and tinned foods, most of which have high additive content. Nearly always her lunch will consist of bread snacks such as sandwiches, rolls or pizza etc. Sometimes for a change she treats herself to a chocolate bar, or three (she craves chocolate).

Almost everything she eats has added sugar, all adding to her Candida problem.

To prove my point I should like to draw your attention to a list of symptoms attributed to menopause, which also occur in Candida

Agitation	Blurred and fluctuating vision
Crying without real reason	Depression
Extremely heavy menstruation	Fatigue
Flushing and sweats	Insomnia
Irritability	Jittery behavior
Lack of concentration	Lack of libido
Lethargy	Loss of balance, dizziness
Loss of confidence	Mood swings
Nervous exhaustion	Palpitations
Panic attacks, terror or fright	Persistent headaches
PMS even after cessation of menses	Poor memory
Spots in vision	Unexplained tingling, skin crawls
Vaginal itching, burning or soreness	Weird, spacey feelings

In her book, "Life Change," Dr. B. Evans says, "Women not of European extraction complain less and appear to suffer least from the effects of menopause." Also "Women who suffer from P.M.S. are most likely to find the menopause troublesome." Analyzing those two statements leads to the conclusion that diet and lifestyle play an important role.

So what is the answer to menopause misery? Doctors will offer tranquilizers or H.R.T. Will they help? I know they don't. Tranquilizers may give temporary relief but will only lead to further chemical overload. H.R.T. will cause, or add to, a Candida problem.

Herbs and quality foods have helped women for centuries, let them help you, then your latter years will become a pleasure. (See Ways of Avoiding Drugs).

"With loving care, the change can be made"

MENSTRUATION

Because the immune system is closely linked with hormones, Candida, M.E. and allergies can severely disrupt a woman's menstrual cycle. As hormonal levels fluctuate alarmingly, the timing can be affected and periods can become painful, irregular and abnormally heavy, or stop entirely. Some think they have become pregnant because of missing several months, then suddenly they have to cope with flooding. Others may have a period every two or three weeks instead of the usual twenty eight days. Almost anything can happen.

Endometriosis, a condition in which the wall of the womb becomes hardened, can be a result of uncontrolled Candida activity and can become serious enough to necessitate a hysterectomy, but if the programme is followed carefully, this can be avoided. As your general health improves, menstrual difficulties will fade, although you must not expect normality for at least six months.

Whatever your menstrual problems are, please go to your doctor and undergo tests to make sure there are no more sinister causes. When you have negative results to your tests you can rule out, and stop worrying about cancer. Set your mind at rest and concentrate on keeping to the programme. Nature will take over.

There are a number of remedies to help you with hormone imbalances. Two or three drops of fennel oil in a glass of spring water twice daily can do wonders. A herb called agnus castus has been known to women for centuries as being able to help with their 'courses' as Culpepper calls them. A blend of agnus castus, magnesium, potassium and vitamin B6 will give wonderful results. Most herbal treatments need to be taken for at least three months to allow them to be absorbed into the system and achieve results, so don't give up on them too soon.

If you have difficulty finding them, call the clinic and we will help.

"Courses need not be curses"

MOULDS

Everyone should be aware of the detrimental affect moulds can have on their health. Living in damp, mouldy accommodation can be a major cause of Candida. Let's analyze just why moulds cause health problems.

Candida albicans is a fungus, moulds are also fungi. The two are closely related in a biological sense because both have asexual means of reproduction. They are, according to one dictionary definition:- 'variously coloured coatings that form on decaying foods. Mildew'.

Food moulds are the least likely to cause problems because we scrape them off or throw the food away. However the mildew mentioned above is a very different problem. Insidiously, it creeps up on us before we are aware of its existence, developing on fabrics, paper, paint and leather. It perpetuates itself throughout the home causing serious allergic reactions.

The problem is that moulds and mildew reproduce by means of spores. Spores are minute air-born particles, rarely visible to the human eye. We both ingest and inhale them. Once inside the body they find perfect conditions to thrive. It is dark and damp and warm. Now they are in a position to cause havoc to our health.

Consider the most common places for moulds to accumulate. Fridges if not kept switched on, around badly sealed sinks, and baths, washbasins and the bottom of shower curtains. Houseplants can also be mould infested, both the leaves and the soil. Change the soil regularly and seal the tops with granite chippings. In fact, anywhere in the home that dampness occurs should be regularly inspected for moulds and mildew. Old houses with cellars are particularly vulnerable. Mould can even be growing in the walls. (Particularly after flooding.)

If you are experiencing severe allergic reactions and you suspect mould in your home is the cause, what can you do?

Arrange to stay away from home for about a week. If you improve, you know your suspicions are right and drastic action must be taken to make your home safe for you.

Scrub the walls with household bleach, make sure piles of discarded clothing and old newspapers are destroyed. Redecorate, sealing walls and treating with an anti-fungicide before fresh paper and paint is applied. Be careful not to breath in either the anti-fungicide chemicals or the spores from old plaster and decorations. Severely allergic people would do well to move out until work is completed.

You could also contact a builder and have him check if there is a structural reason for your home becoming damp and mouldy. He may know of a way to cure the problem.

Paraffin heaters should be avoided because they cause condensation and damp, but a dehumidifier can be helpful to dry out damp corners.

In his book, "The Five Day Allergy Relief System" (Arrow books) Dr. Marshall Mandell tells of an effective way of treating the entire home with formaldehyde. It must be used with great caution because so many people have reacted badly to formaldehyde. However, if proper precautions are observed, this method might prove useful in extreme cases. Full instructions can be found on pages 232-234 of the book.

If all these methods to control moulds fail, then sadly you should consider moving. Your health is the most valuable thing you own and whilst moving can be expensive, moulds could cost you your life.

"We are all a little mouldy,
but some of us are mouldier than others"

MUSCLES - Pains and Cramps

Muscular pain and cramps can be very distressing symptoms and in long periods of immobility, muscle wasting can occur. Try to be as mobile as possible, but *never overwork or stress aching muscles, long term damage may result.*

If you find it truly impossible to exercise, try flexing and relaxing your muscles as you lie in bed or sit in a chair. Start by curling up your toes and clenching your fists. Literally screw yourself up tight, then let it all go limp, breathing in as you tense, and out as you relax, both to a count of four. The clenching will look after your muscles and the breathing will benefit your lungs and oxygenate your blood, as though you were actually doing some form of aerobic exercise. Do it as often as you can. Stop when it hurts, and have another go later. A little and often, is better than making yourself exhausted.

You may find the deep breathing makes you dizzy, don't worry, it is a normal reaction to extra oxygen. If you can do the simple exercise above, you will ease your pain and keep your muscles strong until you are well enough to do more.

Muscle pain will respond well to alternating hot and cold compresses. An easy way is to first apply a hot water bottle, wrapped in a towel to the affected area, then remove it and apply a packet of frozen peas from the freezer. Three minutes with each until the pain abates.

Those are things you can do for yourself, but there is no substitute for loving hands to massage and soothe the pain. If you can't persuade a friend or relative to do it for you, but you can afford to, get a professional masseur to give you a regular treatment.

Check you are not eating something that disagrees with you, allergy can be a reason for muscle pain. Vega testing or Applied Kinesiology will identify the culprit.

"Be like Popeye - Eat up your spinach"

NYSTATIN

This is the most well known of the anti fungal drugs. It was advocated in all the early writings about Candida overgrowth and is still prescribed by doctors. However clinic experience has shown that polyene antibiotics, of which Nystatin is one, actually stimulate the yeasts over an extended period and helps to increase the number of colonies. (See "The Yeast Syndrome" by John Parks Trowbridge, M.D. and Morton Walker, D.P.M. Published by Bantam pages 49-50)

Patients who have been treated with Nystatin come to me two years afterward because their situation was worse than before any form of treatment was given them. Initially they gained remission from their symptoms, only to have them return later. Their eventual condition becomes worse than before. So, following this, the only option left to them, is to be treated by natural medicine and instead of taking 6 to 8 months to improve, it now takes 2 to 3 years.

Nystatin is not the only anti-fungal drug available to doctors. Others are Nizoral, Diflucan, and Fungalin, all of which immediately kill the Candida, but still do not address the real problems, the deficiency of 'friendly flora' in the alimentary tract, a lifetime of bad eating habits and disastrous doctoring methods. Only when the patient understands the causes and changes his lifestyle and eating patterns can the problem be truly overcome.

It also leaves the immune system weak, therefore the patient is open to invasion by any passing 'bugs' and all manner of disease.

There have also been serious reactions to these drugs and unpleasant side effects recorded. This should warn us against there use.

I can't help comparing it to using abortion as a form of birth control. A quick way out of a difficult situation, with no regard for the safety of the patient, later consequences, or teaching of a better way.

*"The better way, is the safe way,
use it to regain quality health"*

OPERATIONS - Surgical

During the course of these illnesses (Candida and M.E.), other unconnected health problems may arise and a surgical operation may be advised. First make absolutely sure it is necessary to have it *now.* If it isn't imperative, put it off until you are considerably better, then with a stronger immune system you will have a better chance of a speedy recovery.

You should also consider how you may react to the anaesthetic, and how long it will remain in your system, making you feel worse. Yes, if you can postpone it, do so. Time may take care of the problem anyway. It is possible that your latest health problem is connected to the immune deficiency and will improve with the treatment you are using without the aid of a knife.

However, you must be sensible. If you have a life threatening condition then you **MUST** do something about it immediately. You can address the M.E., Candida or allergy problem afterwards, at least you will be alive to do so.

Just be wise and ask questions. Be sure there is no other way than to have the surgery and that you are not being subjected to unnecessary treatment because it's the only way they know of dealing with the problem. I know of many people who have avoided operations by using alternative means. Be informed about all possibilities before you agree to undergo surgery.

"Opt out"

PAIN

Pain should never be dismissed or deadened with pain killers until the cause is known. It can be there to draw attention to the site of an illness. The cause must be traced and if possible put right. Nobody finds it easy to tolerate pain, but sometimes it can be an indication of healing taking place.

Once you are satisfied you know the cause, and everything possible has been done to alleviate the reason for it, then is the time to do your best to relieve it. I have mentioned previously the hot/cold compress technique. (See heading "Muscles.") but sometimes cold alone will help. It is always best to try to relieve pain without drugs if possible. When every other method has been exhausted, then and only then should be the time to turn to synthetic preparations, but it must always be remembered that all synthetically prepared painkillers have side effects. Paracetomol for instance, can damage the kidneys.

Herbalists know the value of white willow which is the original form of aspirin, for those with long standing painful conditions there is an amino acid called d'phenylalanine, a natural substance that stimulates production of endomorphins, the body's own pain defences. It is a long term solution because it is about two weeks before it takes effect. Another very useful way of reducing pain is the TENS machine. The abbreviation stands for Transcutaneous Electrical Nerve Stimulation. It delivers minute electrical currents to the nerves at the site of the pain, giving immediate local relief and at the same time stimulating the body to begin producing its own pain relieving hormones. Shaped like a pen, it is light and easy to carry in a pocket or handbag. Use it anywhere.

Low back pain is common in people who have colonic disturbances. Regular massage with aromatherapy oils will help if performed skillfully.

Food allergies can be a cause of pain. If you suffer more after eating certain foods, cut them out of your diet.

"You will gain by reducing your pain"

PREGNANCY

Pregnancy should be one of the most delightful experiences of a woman's life. Unfortunately for Candida and M.E. sufferers this is not the case, although some allergy sufferers gain respite from reactions during pregnancy.

In the first few months of pregnancy, women find their energy levels plummet, along with nausea and morning sickness. Imagine how much worse these symptoms become if you are already ill before you become pregnant. One lady told me it was a waking nightmare for her, and confessed she had seriously considered suicide, only abstaining for the sake of her unborn child. There are varying stages of misery depending on the initial health condition of the mother.

For those anxious to have a child, there are many things to consider. If you are feeling dreadful now, how will you be with another human being dependent on you for everything? Babies are demanding of both time and energy, have you enough to survive? If you have none now, what sort of life can you hope to make for a child until you are well? What health heritage can you pass on? Only what you have yourself is passed to offspring. If you are sick, you will probably give birth to a sickly, ailing child.

Another thing to take into account is, if you currently suffer from thrush, how much of it will pass to your baby as it travels through the birth canal. You know how you are suffering, do you want to condemn your child to a similar experience.

The last thing to consider is the quality of your breast milk. If your body is short of the bifidus bifodum bacterium, so essential for the formation of healthy digestion and immunity, then you may rob your child of a healthy heritage. Add to all this the fact that unhealthy babies are unhappy babies, who cry day and night, and you will agree it might be wiser to wait until you are well before trying to conceive.

All that is bad news, but the good news is, if you are prepared to work hard on the programme for a few months you can have a happy, healthy, comfortable pregnancy, leading to a wonderful bouncing baby.

For those who find themselves pregnant without planning, you must make the best of it. You can help yourself considerably. Immediately you know you are pregnant, begin taking extra probiotic supplementation to ensure supplies to the unborn child during the pregnancy and afterwards, your breast milk will be rich in it.

Make sure you have adequate rest in the day and sleep at night. It is much more important for you than for the average pregnant woman. Try to avoid noisy, smoky atmospheres, they too can badly affect you and your unborn baby. Stick scrupulously to your anti Candida diet and supplement plan right through. It would be wise to consult a nutritionist at least once a month until baby is born.

When your baby finally comes into the world, give him a daily supplement of bifidus infantis. You will have then done everything in your power to give your child the best possible start.

If you have been longing to start a family and have failed to become pregnant, Candida could be the reason. When Candida is cleared, pregnancy follows easily. Just be patient and wait until you're well, and a normal conception and birth will be yours. (See letter on pages 107/8).

What is more, you will be the really proud parent of a lovely healthy baby.

"Sons are a gift from the Lord
and children are a reward from Him"
Psalms 127 v 3

PROBIOTICS

This is the name given to the helpful bacteria that inhabits the human gut. The word means 'for life'. They are sometimes referred to as 'friendly flora' simply because they really are just that, friendly living organisms. Think of them as the 'good guys'. The cavalry employed by the body to keep the 'baddies' under control. Whilst there are many different strains, the treatment of Candida and allergy usually requires only two, bifidus bifodum and Lactobaccilus acidophilus. It is important to know that they establish themselves in the order I have mentioned them in the alimentary tract. ***They are vital to good health,*** maintaining a balance and holding back invasion of harmful bacteria and parasites.

However in some instances, for some people with M.E. seven strains used synergistically in a complex form are beneficial. At the clinic we have developed a special mix. It is called PB7. Sadly it is only available from the clinic direct, but we shall be happy to post it to you if you contact us at the address in the back of this book. (See "Useful Addresses")

Bifidus bifodum should be established first as it is the predominant probiotic found in breast milk. Its purpose is to line the digestive tract of the infant and create strong immunity. You may know, breast fed babies do not contract the ailments of the rest of the family whilst they are being suckled. It has been noted also that babies deprived of breast feeding frequently have bowel disorders. It is necessary to use bifidus at the very start of treatment, because you can't improve on nature. It will not only do for you what it does for babies, but if you have bowel irregularities it will put them right.

L. acidophilus, does not join bifidus in the gut until a child is between five and seven years old, or until weaning is totally complete. When these two are well established in the alimentary tract the immune system is fully operational to face exposure to the germs that assail us throughout life. ***It is important to follow the same sequence nature uses if we intend to rebuild immunity.***

Those who need the multi-strain product would also use it as the second probiotic in their course of treatment, except in exceptional cases determined by a practitioner.

Each time antibiotics, hormones or steroids are used, the careful balance of probiotics comes under attack. *The flora MUST be replaced if you are to regain your health.* If a life threatening health problem does arise, making it imperative for you to take any of these medications to preserve your life, then please take the mix of seven strains at the same time, and for a week or so afterward to keep your immunity strong. A serious asthma attack might be such a time.

Probiotics are a major part of your supplement programme. **NEVER TAKE THEM WITH TAP WATER.** Chlorine is added to destroy bacteria and it will kill your supplement before you even swallow it.

You should select your probiotics with great care. There are a wide variety on the market, and great claims are made. They vary in efficiency from totally useless, to exactly right for your needs. A good rule is to find one with the highest number of viable live organisms per teaspoonful (if in powder form) or per capsule. Encapsulation costs extra money in the manufacturing, so to keep costs down choose quality powders if possible.

When buying multi-strain products, be cautious because some may contain a strain called streptoccocus faecium. There has been speculation as to whether this bacteria remains harmless if allowed to escape through the gut wall to other sites in the body where it might become pathogenic, (meaning capable of causing disease). Since many of those suffering from candidiasis will have a 'leaky gut', they must be alerted to the possible risk.

"Buy carefully, buy well and be well"

PROGRESS

In long term illnesses, progress seems interminable slow. It is made worse by the fact that we live in a world used to modern 'miracle' drugs. Take one at 10am and by 2pm you are fine. Real healing doesn't come about like that, it is a slow but sure progression. Sometimes hardly noticeable.

Whatever you are suffering from, those around you, and possibly you yourself may believe 'they' can give you something to make you better tomorrow, or the next day at the very latest. Unfortunately there really is nothing much to speed things up in this case. You must get used to the fact, *it is going to take time.*

Your immune system, as I explained under the last heading "Probiotics," has taken years to fully develop and probably longer to be destroyed. You have to rebuild it. There is only one really successful way. *Naturally.* There are no shortcuts if you want to be well for the rest of your life.

All who are familiar with complementary medicine will be aware natural healing often means two steps forward and one back. Your body can and will do it if you give it the right building blocks. They are diet, supplements, rest and *time.* Try to be patient.

"Patients with patience WILL make progress"

QUESTIONS

Every individual has a multitude of questions. Some of them are common to most people, so this book has been compiled and designed to answer the questions I have been asked repeatedly throughout my years in practice.

It can never be totally complete and comprehensive because conditions change, supplements improve, knowledge advances but above all people are all individuals, with symptoms, case histories and worries uniquely their own.

If you have a question that is not covered, or that this book fails to answer for you, please write it down and send it to the publisher. It will be passed on to me and I shall do my best to answer it for you, but please enclose a stamped addressed envelope.

This will not only help you, but it will enable me to include it in further editions and updates of this book to help other readers.

"Why me?"

REACTIONS

If you break your diet, after only a short time you could have quite severe reactions. People ask me what these are likely to be. It is very difficult to specify because no two people react in precisely the same way to a given allergen.

The reaction can happen within a few minutes or anytime up to 48 hours later, varying in intensity from slightly irritating to life threateningly severe. I have known people with a milk allergy have some cream on a sweet whilst out to dinner, and within minutes, come out in an embarrassing rash. Another person doing the same thing could be rushed to hospital and put in an oxygen tent with a severe, life threatening asthma attack.

Really there is no definite answer to what will happen to you if if you break the rules. What is certain is, you should know your own body and be aware of what your particular allergens are, and what symptoms they cause. The thought of a reaction may be a good deterrent from breaking your diet.

If you do disregard your body's warnings, you must be warned that not only could you suffer nasty reactions, but you will also cause the programme a set back and waste all the money you have spent on supplements. A reaction will set you back quite a way.

Of course there are some substances that cause reactions over which you have no control. Air pollution is one and chemical and agricultural sprays are others. Cigarette smoke and perfume in public places can be extremely hazardous for some. These are only a few of the problems causing sufferers untold stress. The advice under the heading "Allergies, living with them" will be of help to you in avoiding as many reactions as possible. The only real answer is to keep working on your immune system until it is strong enough to cope with all the allergens surrounding everyone.

"Perseverance pays off"

READING MATTER

There are a number of books about Candida, but very little of any usefulness has been written about M.E. probably because orthodox medicine has shrouded it in mystery. The press, at first made much of it but when no 'instant' cures were forthcoming from the world of drugs, they lost interest. This is not very helpful to sufferers because if the cause remains a 'mystery' so does the cure.

Alternative medicine however, has quietly and progressively applied the basic rules of the natural approach and begun to make valuable breakthroughs. The programme set out in this book has been extremely successful in restoring M.E. sufferers to good health. Unfortunately the treatment is not of the 'magic bullet' variety, so does not make for good press copy.

Nevertheless complementary practitioners are helping, and some of them are committing their findings and treatments to the written page to help sufferers to find solutions.

To this end, in Britain, there are two groups who publish information for Candida and M.E. sufferers. They offer membership on a small subscription basis. They are:-

Interaction Journal, published by Action for M.E. and Chronic Fatigue. P.O., Box 1302, Wells, Somerset. BA5 2WE. Tel 01749 670799

The National Candida Society, P.O. Box 151, Orpington, Kent, BR5 1UJ. www.candidasociety.org.uk

Both organizations are well intended and offer information, advice and support, endeavoring to keep members up to date with latest medical thinking. As I write, The National Candida Society has begun trials on two anti-fungal herbs. It would be good to have a greater variety of remedies that could be relied upon to achieve results, as some people may react unfavorably to some medication. We must await results. No doubt the results will be published when they are known.

Reading too much on the subject can be confusing as each author has his or her own opinions on the subject and the advice given differs. In the end the reader doesn't know what course of action to take and despairingly decides to do nothing for fear of getting it wrong. Because of this I recommend only three books. They are:-

1) "Candida albicans, Yeast and Your Health" by Gill Jacobs. Published by Optima. Well researched information, collated and presented in an unbiased way.

2) "The Yeast Syndrome" by John Parks Trowbridge and Morton Walker Published by Bantam. An American publication presenting extensive research and the latest expertise in the American field.

3) "Candida albicans. Could Yeast be your problem?" by Leon Chaitow. Published by Thorsons. Dr. Chaitow has followed the development of probiotic treatments from the start. He has consistently updated his book to take into account new developments.

All these are available by post from Foyles book shop, London.
(See useful addresses).

If you find extensive reading difficult because of your health, you will find "Candida M.E. and Allergies - The Way Back to Good Health," is very comprehensive and includes information not to be found elsewhere. It has been enough, since it was first published to help 1000s of people back to good health.

"As regards anything besides these my son,
take a warning:
to the making of many books there is no end and
much devotion to them is wearisome to the flesh."
Ecc 12 v 12.

RECIPES

These are just a few useful recipes to bring a little more variety to the basic diet. No doubt, in time, you will develop and collect more of your own. You may also find my book 'Cooking for Candida' useful.

Bean Burgers

250gm (8oz) aduki or kidney beans
2 sticks celery, chopped small
1 large onion, chopped small
2 teaspoons mixed herbs
1 or 2 cloves garlic, crushed
2 teaspoons yeast free stock powder
1 free range egg
pepper to taste

Method
Mix all the ingredients together and mold into shapes (if mixture is too wet add a little rice or potato flour). Roll the burger in oatmeal and set in the fridge to firm. Fry in olive oil and serve hot with vegetables or a mixed salad.

Basic Cheese Sauce

500ml (1 carton) soya milk
1 tablespoon corn flour
100g (4ozs) vegetarian cheese

Method
Mix corn flour with a little of the milk, heat rest of milk in a pan. Add corn flour and grated cheese, stirring until thickened.

This is good on cauliflower with fish (if not wheat sensitive with pasta). Cold without the cheese makes good blancmange, but add more corn flour and a little fructose after the first month Without the cheese, this method will make a basic sauce to which you can add almost anything.

Chicken Supreme

125g (4ozs) whole grain brown rice
500ml (1pint) carton soya milk
diced fresh vegetables of choice
1 teaspoon corn flour
leftover cooked chicken (this works well with prawns too)

Method
Boil rice with veg and a few herbs until soft. Stand aside. Make basic white sauce as above. Add chicken pickings. Drain rice and make nest on plate, pour the sauce in centre.

This dish turns into an acceptable curry when curry powder is added to the sauce.

Nut and Seed Roast

1 cup shelled nuts
1 cup sunflower seeds
1 cup sesame seeds
½ cup pumpkin seeds
1 onion-finely chopped
3 cloves-finely chopped
½ green pepper
1 tsp pepper
1 tsp tomato purée
1 tsp mixed herbs
olive oil for frying

Method
Preheat oven to 220°C (425°F) Gas 7. Blend all nuts and seeds together to form a bread crumb texture. Chop onion finely and fry in olive oil, adding garlic and pepper at the same time. Blend in all other ingredients except tomato purée and nut mixture. Cook until onions are golden

brown. Now add brown nut mixture stirring well, all the time, to prevent it sticking to the pan. Only cook until mixture is well blended, otherwise the nuts could burn.

Make a tomato juice with 1 cup boiling water and the tomato purée.

Put the fried ingredients into a loaf tin and pour on the tomato juice, until a sloppy mixture is formed. Cook for about 40 minutes until top is well browned. 200° C (400° F) Gas 6.

Curried Cod

450g (1lb) cod
50g (2ozs) marg (whey free)
1 onion sliced
1 clove garlic
1 tablespoon organic flour or cornflour
1 level dessert spoon curry powder
½ litre (1pint) fish or chicken stock
salt

Method
Set oven at 180°C (350°F) or Gas 4. Cut cod into 4cm (1½") squares. Mix salt with flour and dip cod pieces into this mixture. Melt half marg into frying pan and quickly fry fish until golden brown, but not cooked through. Place fish in a casserole. Put rest of marg in pan, add onion and garlic and cook until golden brown, sprinkle in curry powder and any flour left over from coating fish, then cook for 2 mins. Remove from heat and stir in stock, a little at a time. Return to heat and bring to boil. Pour this sauce over fish and cook in oven for 20 mins. Serve with plain boiled rice.

Oriental Lamb   (Serves 4) Not during the 1st month of diet

450g (1lb) lean diced lamb
1 tbs dried mint
2 large onions, peeled and sliced
225g (8ozs) long grain rice
625ml (1¼ pints) stock
salt and pepper
2 courgettes topped, tailed and cut into diagonal pieces
225g (8ozs) can dried peach or apricot halves in natural juice
50g (2ozs) baby corn on the cob trimmed

Method
In a large frying pan, gently fry lamb by itself until meat starts to brown. Add mint and toss for 2 mins, stirring continuously. Add meat and bring to the boil. Reduce heat, cover pan and simmer gently for 30-35 mins. Stir in courgettes, peaches and corn. Re-cover and cook for a further 10-15 mins or until rice has absorbed the liquid and the meat is tender. Serve hot with crisp green salad.

Tuna Fish Bake
basic white sauce (see page 145)
1 tin of tuna (drain the brine)
salt and pepper
crushed potato crisps (salt & veg oil only)
can of sweet corn (drained)

Method
Mix tuna in the white sauce, top with crisps and sweet corn, bake in moderate oven for about 45 mins. 200° C (400° F) Gas 6.

Serve hot with green salad.

Yeast Free Bread   For those who can tolerate wheat

575g (1lb 4oz) brown organic self raising flour
2 free range eggs
2 teaspoons of salt or substitute
soya milk

Method
Preheat the oven with the baking tray in it whilst making the dough. Sift the flour and salt together. Beat eggs with milk and add a little water. Make a 'well' in the flour and gradually add the egg mixture, using the hands to combine the ingredients and to form a soft pliable but not wet dough. The dough should clean the bowl of the flour without being too sticky. Knead the dough on a floured surface for a few minutes, then flatten to form a large circle about 30cm (12 inches) diameter. Score the bread down the centre and across with a knife as in a hot cross bun. Put into a hot oven on a floured baking tray 220° C (425° F) Gas 7 and bake for 10 minutes. Turn bread over. Continue baking until the bread has been in the oven for half an hour. When cooked, the bread can be cut where scored and frozen if necessary. This is a dry bread and needs plenty of vegetable margarine. You may also form rolls and freeze until needed.

If the bread is cooked through it will sound hollow when tapped.

Almond and Soya Biscuits
225g (½lb) ground almonds
800g (4lbs) soya flour
2 free range egg yolks
water to mix

Method
Put almond flour into bowl. Add 2 tablespoons water to egg yolks then add to flour. Form into sausage, cut into slices and bake on oiled tray 220°C (425°F) Gas 7 for about 20 minutes until light golden brown.

Polenta

275g (10oz) maize flour
2 teaspoons salt
750ml (1½ pints) water (or half soya milk and half water)
an optional extra 2 teaspoons mixed herbs for a savoury flavour

Method
Put water, flour and salt into large pan. Stirring constantly, bring to the boil and boil for 2 minutes until it thickens. Pour into greased roasting tin and bake 190°C (375°F) Gas 5 for an hour or until firm enough to turn when cool. When cold, slice and grill or fry. Lovely with fried egg omelette and salad.

Chick Pea Flour (Gram flour) biscuits

450g (1lb) chick pea flour
2 free range egg yolks
water to mix
poppy seeds

Method
Put flour into a bowl. Make a 'well' in the centre. Add 5 tbs water to egg yolks. Mix, then mix in the flour to a kind of pastry. If to wet, add more flour. Form into a ball. Cut into 3 sections. Roll out each section using more chick pea flour and cut into biscuit shapes as thinly as possible. Bake on oiled tray 220°C (425°F) Gas 7 for about 20 minutes until light golden brown.

Sunflower Wedge

1 cup carrots and 1 cup celery, finely chopped
½ teaspoon salt
1 teaspoon basil
50g (1½oz) dairy free margarine
cup sunflower seeds
½ cup oatmeal
sesame seeds (toasted)

Method
Combine all ingredients and press into a 20 cm (8") sandwich tin. Mark out into sections. Cook at 180°C (350°F) Gas 4 for about 1 hour. Halfway through cooking, sprinkle with the sesame seeds (press in). Keep in fridge. Freezes well.

Buckwheat Pancakes   (For those who cannot tolerate wheat)

125g (4oz) buckwheat flour
1 free range egg
salt and pepper
soya or goat milk

Method
Make up the batter by adding an egg to dry ingredients. Then add enough milk to make a smooth batter.

Fry pancakes and fill with your hearts desire (but within the rules), try tuna or sweet corn leftovers. For a sweet treat, try apple concentrate poured over.

Home Made Mayonaise

1 free range egg
2 tablespoons lemon juice
1 cup olive oil
1 teaspoon mustard (optional)
¼ teaspoon powdered kelp (optional)
¼ teaspoon salt (optional)

Method
Blend, dribble oil down the back of a fork a little at a time as you beat the rest of the ingredients.

Hummus

50g (2oz) chick peas soaked and boiled then mashed, blend in 1 tablespoon Tahini (sesame seed paste available at health shops, delicatessens), 1 clove crushed garlic and the juice of a lemon. Blend well adding water if necessary to achieve smooth thick cream. Use on salad as a dressing or as a dip with raw veg made into sticks, celery is terrific and so are carrots.

Carrot Cake

225g (8oz) carrot puréed
4 free range egg yolks
175g (6oz) ground almonds or ground hazelnuts

Method
Beat egg yolks and add to carrot purée then add ground nuts. Put into oiled cake tin and bake for 50 minutes at 200°C (400°F) Gas 6. This cake should be refrigerated or cut into slices and frozen then taken out as needed.

Lentil Cake

8 oz lentils
2 free range egg yolks
a little oil

Method
Simmer lentils after soaking for about an hour in stock or water. They should not be to sloppy. When mixture has boiled a little, add egg yolks and a little oil. Transfer to oiled loaf tin. Bake at 220°C (425°F) Gas 7 for 45 minutes. The top should be crunchy. It can be eaten in slices hot, or toasted under the grill when cold. This cake does not keep, so should also be refrigerated. Mixed herbs or other seasonings can be added according to taste.

Sunflower Seed Biscuits

1¼ tablespoons sunflower seeds ground
3 tablespoons carrot, cooked and puréed
2 or 3 free range egg yolks

Method
Put sunflower seeds in a large bowl reserving 4 tablespoons of the flour for shaping the loaf. Add egg yolks to carrot purée and then mix into flour. Shape into a long sausage or loaf shape using reserved flour. Cut into slices and bake on oiled tray until brown. These biscuits need turning. Bake at 220°C (450°F) Gas 7 for about 20 minutes.

Yummy Come Again Cake

1 cup brown rice flour
½ cup oil
2 teaspoons baking powder
2 teaspoons vanilla essence
1 teaspoon ground ginger
2 heaped teaspoons mixed spice
2 medium sized carrots (grated)

Method
Beat all ingredients together and place mixture in a greased 18cm (7")
cake tin, (preferably with a removable bottom). Cook in a medium oven
until risen and golden brown. Serve hot with margarine and mixed spice
sprinkled on top, or your favourite spread. You can substitute any fruit
allowable on your personal diet. Apple or banana is particularly good.

Oatmeal Muffins Without flour

4 cups rolled oats
½ teaspoon salt substitute
2 teaspoons salt free baking powder
3 free range eggs
1 cup goat or sheep milk
5 tablespoons sunflower oil

Method
Liquidize (blend oats until powdery), add salt substitute and baking
powder. Beat eggs in separate bowl. Combine in blender 1 cup luke-
warm milk and the sunflower oil, add this to the egg yolks and then fold
in flour mixture. Mix quickly and pour into muffin or cake tins. Bake
25 minutes 220°C (425°F) Gas 7 until firm. If the muffins are to damp
in the middle I usually cut them in half and then bake for a few minutes
to dry off.

Rice and Oat Muffins

1 cup oatmeal
¾ cup rice flour (sifted)
3 teaspoons baking powder
½ teaspoon salt
¾ cup milk (soya)
1 free range egg

Method
Preheat the oven to 180°C (350°F) Gas 4. Grease muffin tray. Mix flour, baking powder and salt then mix in remaining ingredients. Pour into tray and bake for approximately 25 minutes. Cut muffins in half and spread with desired topping.

Scones

225g (8ozs) rice flour
2 teaspoons baking powder
50g (2ozs) vegetarian margarine
1 free range egg
75ml (2fl ozs) soya milk

Method
Sift flour and baking powder together and rub in margarine. Mix to a dough with lightly beaten egg and milk. Cut into rounds and put onto greased baking sheet. Brush lightly and bake for 15-20 minutes, 220°C (425°F) Gas 7. These scones are better with vegetarian cheese added.

Carrot Cookies

1 cup brown rice flour
2 medium carrots (grated)
6 dessert spoons oil
6 dessert spoons water
1 teaspoon baking powder
2 teaspoons vanilla essence
mixed spice or ginger according to taste

Combine all ingredients and roll into balls in hands, press out on floured board and arrange on greased baking sheet. Cook until brown, for about 10 to 15 minutes 220°C (425°F) Gas 7.

Mung Bean Biscuits

1 bag mung bean flour
2 free range egg yolks
4 tablespoons puréed cooked carrot

Method
Put flour into mixing bowl. Add egg yolks to carrot and then to mixture. As before, reserve a little flour for shaping into sausage or loaf shape. Cut into slices and bake on oiled tray until brown. These biscuits need turning. Bake at 220°C (425°F) Gas 7 for about 20 minutes.

RECIPES THAT INCLUDE FRUIT FOR AFTER THE FIRST MONTH

Moroccan Rice Salad
175g (6ozs) brown rice,
2 bananas, sliced
½ cucumber
2 tablespoons raisins
1 tablespoon sliced almonds
4 tablespoons olive oil
4 tablespoons lemon juice
½ teaspoon ground cumin
½ teaspoon cayenne pepper
1 teaspoon sea salt

Method
Cook the rice, drain and allow to cool, add the bananas, cucumber, raisins and sliced almonds and mix well together.
Place all the other ingredients in a screw topped jar and shake well together. Pour the dressing over the rice mixture, toss and serve.

You may add other fruit and vegetables, pumpkin seeds and sunflower seeds, anything you fancy to ring the changes to this basic rice dish. In a sealed container, it is very good to take for lunches when away from home.

Orange Oat Cookies
75g (3ozs) dairy free margarine
1 orange (chopped small or put in food processor)
50g (2ozs) wholemeal or rice flour
25g (1oz) ground almonds
25g (1oz) porridge oats

Method
Soften the margarine and beat in orange. Mix in all other ingredients. Put a teaspoon of mixture on a greased baking sheet, allowing room to

Apple Cake

50g 2ozs rice flour
50g 2ozs soya flour
4ozs potato flour
6ozs margarine
2 free range eggs
2 teaspoons baking powder
¼ teaspoon salt
cinnamon
2 cooking apples

Method
Cream margarine and mix with eggs. Fold in flours, baking powder and salt. Put half mixture in greased cake tin. Peel, core and slice apples and lay on top of the mixture and sprinkle with cinnamon. Cover apple with remaining mixture and bake 1½ hours 180°C (350°F) Gas 4.

Apple Crumble

50g (2ozs) rice flour
50g (2ozs) soya flour
50g (2ozs) oats
50g (2ozs) dairy free margarine
450g (1lb) apples

Method
Mix flours and oats and rub in margarine. Put mixture over fruit. Bake 15-20 minutes 190°C (375°F) Gas 5.

Banana Ice cream

Remove skins from 2 bananas and place in freezer, when solid put them in a blender or food processor. (Chop if necessary.) Add ½ cup water and blend until creamy. Eat immediately.

Mousaka

450g (1lb) minced lamb (or beef if top quality)
225g (8ozs) onions, peeled and sliced
3-4 cloves garlic, crushed
2 medium aubergines, cut into rounds approximately ½" thick
2 tablespoons tomato purée
1 teaspoon ground cinnamon
1 tablespoon freshly chopped parsley
olive oil, sea salt and freshly milled black pepper

Topping

(50g) 2ozs flour
(50g) 2ozs dairy free margarine
15fl ozs (¾pint) unsweetened soya milk
50g (1½ozs) vegetarian cheese, grated
1 large free range egg, beaten
sea salt, pepper and freshly ground nutmeg

Method
Preheat oven to 180°C (350°F) gas 4

First prepare the aubergines. Slice, then place in a colander, sprinkle with sea salt, cover with a plate and place something heavy on top to weight it down. This extracts the bitter juices. Leave for 30 minutes.

Fry onions and garlic in olive oil till soft, add minced meat and brown, stirring to break up any lumps. In a basin, mix together tomato purée, cinnamon and parsley, add a little filtered water and salt and pepper.

Pour this mixture into pan with onions and mince, stir well and leave on gentle heat to simmer.

Heat olive oil in a fresh frying pan, rinse and dry aubergine, slice well and fry until golden brown on both sides, remove from pan and drain on kitchen paper (they really soak up the olive oil). Take a casserole dish and arrange layers of aubergines with layers of meat mixture.

Sauce:-
Melt margarine in pan, stir in flour till smooth, add milk gradually stirring well to make a smooth white sauce. Next, stir in the cheese, add salt, pepper and nutmeg. Allow to cool slightly then add the beaten egg and stir well.

Pour the sauce over the meat and aubergine layers, then bake (uncovered) for an hour until the top is fluffy golden.

Quick Pizza

225g (8ozs) organic flour
pinch natural salt
75g (2½ozs) dairy free margarine
150ml (¼pint) unsweetened soya milk
1 large onion, skinned and sliced
200g (7oz) can tomatoes (or skinned fresh tomatoes)
¼ green pepper, sliced into thin strips
1 or 2 cloves of garlic, crushed
1 generous tablespoon of tomato purée
2 pinches dried mixed herbs
175g (6ozs) grated vegetarian cheese to taste

Method
Stir flour and salt into a bowl, then rub in 50g (2ozs) of margarine to form bread crumbs. Add milk and mix to soft dough. Turn onto floured surface and knead until smooth. Roll out to one large shape (to fit tin) about 1.5cm (½inch) thick. Place on greased baking tin or tray. Fry

onions and garlic in remaining margarine. Spread tomato purée onto pizza base, sprinkle lightly with mixed herbs and a little grated cheese. Place onions and garlic on next and top with the tomatoes, seasoning, mixed herbs and grated cheese. Arrange pepper strips on to decorate, with thin slices of tomato if desired. Bake in the oven at 220°C (425°F) Gas 7 for 20-25 minutes until cooked and golden.

Allowable Snacks and Treats
Crisps. Ingredients: only potatoes, salt, vegetable oil, (not hydrogenated)
almonds
blanched almonds
pumpkin seeds
sunflower seeds
mung beans (sprouted)
chick peas (sprouted)
popped corn. Do it yourself in olive oil. Add a little salt.
Tortilla chips
Supermarket nondairy cream

REFLEXOLOGY

Reflexology is a form of massage applied to the feet. It is said to have originated in China some 5000 years ago. It is a means of clearing the 'energy channels' of the body by applying pressure to the feet in the reflex areas. It is useful if the energy flow has become blocked by illness and can bring relief and comfort without resorting to drugs.

I am repeatedly asked, "Will it help?" The true answer is, "It depends what your expectations are." If you are looking for a complete cure from this treatment, then the answer is no, but if you look upon it as a part of a balanced programme aimed at restoring your body to a proper working order, then it can contribute by clearing the energy channels to over stressed organs and giving a sense of balance to the entire energy system.

Practitioners who use this therapy find it an invaluable diagnostic tool. It is also a way to stimulate parts of the body that have become sluggish in order to raise general energy levels.

Yes, providing no extravagant claims are made, or too much expected of it, reflexology can prove of benefit, but, if money is short and a choice of treatments has to be made to suit the pocket, you should never substitute a reflexology treatment for your supplements.

"There is something 'afoot'"

RELAXATION

This is a word translated in many ways by different people. To healthy, energetic folk it could mean an hour on a squash court or a round of golf. To someone who is ill, it may mean the opportunity to sneak into bed for an hour. However we personally understand the word, it most definitely describes what we do with our time when we have a choice.

To some it denotes a floppy condition of the muscles whilst clearing the mind of stress. The ability to do it is quite an art, and wonderfully good for you if you can achieve it. Unfortunately most people have lost the ability. The world we live in 'winds us up' we are like a 'coiled spring' in an over wound clock, totally unable to let go. So for those who would like to relearn the art of relaxation here are a few simple instructions.

Find yourself a quiet place, then clench your fists and screw your face up, so hard you make the muscles in your neck stand out. Tell yourself out loud, *this is tension.* Breath in and hold it for 4 seconds (slowly count to four). Next, slowly exhale letting your whole body go limp and floppy for a further count of 4, at the same time say aloud, *this is relaxation.* Repeat the whole process ten times.

You can do this exercise in bed if you have difficulty sleeping. If you do it often enough, it will impress itself on your subconscious, just the way a 'pop' song does when it is played repeatedly. Before long your brain will be reprogrammed to know the difference and respond automatically when you just think the word, relax. The art of relaxation will become yours again, just as when you were a child and could fall asleep anywhere. Maybe you relax best with a book, watching T.V. or listening to music. Whatever helps you most, reap the rewards relaxation can bring.

"Be 'laid back'"

REST

Never under estimate the value of having enough rest. Some may tell you to keep going, press on regardless. **Rubbish!** If everything in your being is telling you to stop, *do it, take it easy,* sleep if you can. Don't feel guilty about it, guilt has a destructive effect on your health. Listen to your body, and rest as much as you possibly can.

There is an old saying *"Never stand when you can sit, never sit when you can lie down."* In the case of M.E. and Candida sufferers, I endorse it wholeheartedly. I will even add to it..... *"Never walk when you can ride, never stay awake when you could be sleeping."* Rest and sleep are among the most valuable things you can do to help your body heal itself. (See heading on Electromagnetism and M.E.)

A good deal of natural healing takes place whilst you sleep. When you wake up not feeling refreshed it could be because your body needs more sleep in order to complete the repairs needed to your battered immune system. Have you ever noticed how animals creep under a hedge, curl into a ball and sleep when they are unwell? Take a lesson from them.

If people accuse you of being lazy, pay no attention to them, they have no concept of how awful you feel, or how tired just the smallest amount of exertion can make you.

Delegate responsibility, don't take on an extra unnecessary thing that will require action from you. If possible...

"Cancel tomorrow and rest"

SEX

Although the tabloids and television programmes are full of it, the subject of sex is still a difficult one for many decent people to broach. Some have never heard the medical terminology for sex drive, 'libido' and feel the subject is not to be mentioned.

For Candida and M.E. sufferers, their 'libido' is one of the first things to go and last to return. Just the very thought of it makes them feel tired, without actually indulging in intercourse. However, this does not mean sex is out of the question for everyone suffering from these conditions.

Many still retain their ability and enjoyment. What you should be made aware of is that thrush can be transmitted through intercourse, to your partner. You could toss it back and forth between you continuously unless you are both treated and cleared of it simultaneously.

Men can infect partners if they carry it round the groin or under the foreskin. Women, with vaginal thrush can likewise pass it on. So, if you plan to indulge, and lets face it, your life could do with a little excitement and brightening up, do be responsible about it. Take precautions against infecting your partner. If you have oral thrush, don't kiss your partner on the mouth, if you have it around the genitalia, use a condom.

These are the only two rules, the rest is up to you.

"If you can summon up the energy, have fun"

SMOKING

What a terrible, insidious narcotic, nicotine really is! Of all the 'recreational' drugs commonly indulged in, it is the only one that is so addictive that users have to have a 'fix' between the courses of a meal. I really do feel for anyone trying to break themselves of the habit. I know how hard it was for me to stop, but 'kick it' I did and that was over half a lifetime ago, so I know it can be done.

I shall not say all the obvious things you have no doubt heard it all from others. What you need to understand is, it is imperative you stop smoking if you are to be well.

One, little publicized fact is, *tobacco is cured on sugar. As you take puff after puff, you are inhaling it in large quantities.* It will feed your problem just as fast as if you were taking tablespoonsful in your food at every meal. If you continue to smoke you will nullify all your attempts to free yourself from Candida overgrowth.

Please make a real effort to stop. Something I found of real help to me, was to change the subject in my mind each time I thought of lighting up. It may work for you. You must become aware of what you are doing with your hands because it becomes a reflex. Throw both your mind and your hands into something of interest and the intervals between craving will become longer. If you believe in God, pray for help. As it is such an unclean habit He will be sure to answer. Prayer is doubly powerful, it enlists divine help and at the same time changes the subject in your mind.

For practical, instant help in overcoming the craving for a 'fag' some have found vitamins B complex and C with calcium and magnesium works for them. In sublingual form they will work instantly. Auricular therapy has helped some smokers but best of all is will power.

"Don't send your health up in smoke"

STARTING YOUR PROGRAMME

Step 1) Food Tests

After establishing you really do have Candida or M.E. The first thing to do is to have food tests done to find out the extent of your immune breakdown. This will identify the foods causing you to have allergic reactions. Keep a list of them, not just in order to avoid eating them, although it is important, but also because, as treatment progresses, you will find the number of foods you are reacting to will decrease. This serves as an indicator of how successful you have been in restoring your immune system. It is also an encouragement to see food related symptoms disappearing. Eventually you will be able to reintroduce them, but don't try too soon, immunity takes a long time to recover. Anything from 6 months to 3 years I have found.

Step 2) The Diet

Now, sit down with your food allergy results and the suggested diet in the book, and check that the diet doesn't include any of your personal sensitivities. If necessary, make minor adjustments to suit your own needs. An example might be, you are unable to tolerate onions, so you would delete them from the recipe and substitute with garlic or leeks. When you have completed it, you will have a diet tailored to to fit your individual needs. *Remember this is not a slimming diet,* so eat as much as you like of the foods you can have. You are now more than half way to good health, so let me explain your objectives.

The adjusted diet will help alleviate any allergic reactions, so you will immediately feel brighter. Also, by excluding the foods feeding the Candida, you will stop it multiplying. You are going to starve it to death. Don't be surprised if you find yourself craving sweet foods or alcohol. The craving is set up by the Candida wanting to be fed, death pangs! Don't give in. Your new diet is the first of your weapons to fight not only this dangerous parasite, but your way back to health. You will notice garlic is included regularly in the diet. This is because it's a very effective means of fungal control. Use it at every opportunity.

Step 3) The Supplements
Don't try to cut corners, you need all these things if you are to regain good health
A) An enterically coated anti-fungal agent capable of reaching the colon at full strength. This means a time released product. It must be natural.

B) A really strong strain of bifidus bifodum (approx 30 billion (USA) viable organisms per teaspoonful) This should be taken ½ teaspoonful, twice daily, on an empty stomach, mixed into 250ml (8oz) glass of tepid spring or filtered water. The most effective time to take this is ½ hour before breakfast and last thing before bed. As long after your last meal as possible. After 4 months using bifidus, you should change to L. acidophilus, (again a very powerful strain), first by mixing the two together in 50/50 proportions, then L. acidophilus on its own until you are really well. The time taken to achieve this varies from person to person. The way you feel will let you know when you dare stop taking it, together with freedom from allergies. It is best to reduce dosage over a period of two to three weeks, possibly then continuing on a lower dosage product indefinitely.

C) Now for your daily vitamin needs. These are mega doses to rebuild immunity:-
VitaminA (Betacarotene) 10,500iu
Vitamin E (d-Alfa Tocopherol...195iu
Vitamin C 3,000mg
Vitamin B5 (calcium Pantothenate)..600mg
Magnesium Gluconate.. 300mg
B1 ....104mg
B3 (Nicotinamide) 104mg
B2 ....60mg
Vitamin B6 ....60mg
Inositol...60mg
Choline 60mg
P.A.B.A. 60mg
Zinc Gluconate 60mg
Biotin..4,500mg
Folic Acid 60mg
Vitamin B12 ....60mg
Selenium (Seleniummethionine). 60mg

You will find these precise dosages very expensive to purchase separately, but there are vitamin companies who are combining them into complex products. They should be divided into 3 doses and always taken with food.

Last on your supplement list is the inclusion of garlic and olive oil. Both have been known and used for 1000s of years because of their healing properties.

Garlic for its blood cleansing action, natural antibiotic and anti-fungal qualities. It is also capable of reducing mucous and improves digestion. If you are not able to eat at least 3 cloves a day, raw, then you should include 4 capsules per day, divided in 2 doses, morning and evening with food. It is possible to buy these in deodorised form if you are concerned about the antisocial side effects.

Olive oil as a rich source of oleic acid. It lines the gut and helps your system absorb the other supplements. To gain maximum benefit, it should always be first pressing, virgin oil. Six teaspoons daily is the dose. This can be used on food or made into salad dressing. If for any reason you cant take olive oil, then linseed oil is the next best thing.

For further information about the properties and value of each individual vitamin and mineral included, see the heading "Vitamins."

If you would like help selecting your products, write to me via the publisher and I will send you an up to date list.

" Supplementation spells success"

STOOLS

What is a normal stool? It is difficult to be precise because they vary according to our diet. Meat eaters will find their stools are quite dark and solid, whilst vegetarians can expect lighter and softer texture.

When in Germany I was surprised to discover the toilets had a small shelf to catch them, in order to inspect them before disposal. I am not sure I like the idea, but certainly it is useful to know that what you pass is an indicator of inner health. If you can identify undigested particles of a former meal, you know your digestion needs help. 'Rabbit droppings' would indicate a measure of constipation.

One lady, when she began the programme, reported her stools were like 'cow pats' in vast quantities. This was significant as she had been constipated most of her life. As her colon cleansed itself, her health improved dramatically. It is not unusual to see white flakes or white slime and stringy bits in the stool as treatment progresses. This is a really good sign. It means Candida is dying and being expelled down the drain.

A client who had been fainting whilst passing motions, said she felt better since passing this.... I watched with horror as she unwrapped a parcel.... It contained a piece of white substance about 3 inches across. She had collected it to show me. She had a really serious Candida problem, and the minute she was free of that huge piece, she made rapid progress. I found it hard to imagine how she had passed it. No wonder she had been 'passing out'.

Don't be surprised at the changes to your stools in the first few weeks of treatment, they will settle down to normality when your colon is clean and healthy. You should then pass a comfortable motion at least once or twice daily.

"There is poetry in healthy motions"

STRESS

There are two ways to view stress. Used correctly it can benefit us because it can help us accomplish things we might otherwise be incapable of. To illustrate, imagine yourself peacefully crossing a field, suddenly a bull charges at you. Your eyes see it, your mind registers it and sends an immediate distress signal to your heart. Your heart leaps into action and adrenaline is released into your blood stream. You run for your life, faster than ever before, vault a five bar gate and gain safety.... Stress saved you from calamity.

However, adrenaline releases blood sugar, so it can be disastrous for people with Candida and M.E. The blood sugar feeds their problem from within. A vicious circle.

Highly stressed people are prone to Candida and M.E. and the above is the reason why. They always have an overload of blood sugar because their adrenal glands are continuously activated. If you live your life in a constant state of stress, you will be perpetuating this harmful cycle within yourself. To be well you must break it. Either remove yourself from the causes, or learn to control it from within yourself. Not an easy task. Inner peace is not the gift of us all.

Some people attain it from thoughtful meditation, some from religion, others from yoga or exercise. You have to find the way for you. Search for a way to reduce your stress levels and you will find the way back to good health.

A useful book on the subject is "The Last Straw" by Peter Campbell, published by Arlington Books, London.

"Don't let it get to you"

SUPPLEMENTS

Obtaining your supplements may be a real problem. There are so many to choose from, all claiming great things and varying in price. Sales assistants can be persuasive, but uninformed, or working on commission. A good thing to remember, as with everything else you buy, there is the real thing and cheaper imitations. Make sure you buy the real thing. Many people look at the label and say, 'This is what I want, it has vitamin C, B6, Biotin etc., and it is yeast free, it will do', but will it? Look again. Check the amounts of the ingredients. How many mgs, mcgs or iu's. Find the product to match your exact needs.

If the supplements you buy are not strong enough, you will spend substantial amounts of money and gain no benefit from them. This will mean you will suffer from the symptoms longer, possibly being unfit to work and earn during that period. Not exactly a saving. Mistakes can become very costly indeed, not just in money, but in quality of life.

Over the many years I have been practicing, the most common hurdle to be overcome has been the cost of supplements. This means the quality products that really work, have sometimes been beyond the sufferer's means. If you have this problem ask for expert advice to choose your products. Get the most benefit from the funds you have available to you.

Another problem has been uninformed practitioners, who have recommended various products and treatments that have been unsuccessful. Financial resources are used and the client is no better and now also without funds. Some lose hope that anything can help them and give up.

In Britain, the National Health Service has had the effect of keeping the people totally unaware of the true cost of medication, so the cost of supplements seems to them to be excessive, when in fact they compare very favourably.

I have deliberately omitted the names of products from this

book, because as more research is done, better and more effective supplements will become available. Also, product names change as time passes, and by the time you read this book, much of what I could have written about the availability of supplements might no longer be accurate.

Therefore we at the clinic will endeavor to keep up to date with the latest developments in this field. When you require up to date information about available products simply send a stamped, addressed envelope to me, care of my publisher (See page 1 for the address) and I will be happy to send you a list.

Always remember, you only get what you pay for, so have the best possible supplements within your means. Then you will get the best possible results.

"Your health must have first priority"

SWIMMING

From the time we are very young, water gives us pleasure, and most people progress from paddling and splashing in it, to learning how to swim. We are never too young or too old to enjoy this wonderful relaxing pastime.

Swimming, as well as being pleasurable, is also an excellent form of exercise, especially for those who have muscular problems. It gently works all the muscles at once, not over stressing them, but helping them to keep flexible. As an aerobic exercise it recharges the blood with oxygen and therefore creates more energy.

There is a snag though. The vast majority of swimming pools use heavy applications of chlorine to keep the water free from germs. You must avoid this chemical whilst you are on the programme. Whatever you do, *don't swallow the water.* The added chlorine kills bacteria and you are spending hard earned money trying to repopulate your gut with it, so don't let a swim destroy all the good you have done.

You may find an ozone pool in your locality, if not perhaps a freshwater lake or reservoir, or even the sea (if it is not too polluted in your area).

If your swim has to be taken in a chlorinated pool, please remember to keep your mouth shut...

"Try to keep 'in the swim'"

SYMPTOMS of C.A. and M.E.

The following list of symptoms is rather longer than in other books written on the subject, but has been compiled from the case histories of those I have treated, along with other research.

They all apply to Candida but the ones that are particularly associated with M.E. I have made stand out in **bold** type so that is easy to spot.

GASTRO-INTESTINAL SYSTEM

Abdominal pain
Adhesions *
Chronic heartburn
Colitis *
Diarrhoea
Distension, bloating of abdomen

Excessive gas
Gastritis*
Haemorrhoids (piles)
Indigestion
Mucous in stools
Rectal itching

EARS

Deafness
Excessive wax
Fluid in the ears

Noises
Pain
Recurring infections

EYES

Blurred vision
Burning
Chronic inflammation
Double vision
Erratic vision

Failing vision
Night blindness
Spots on vision
Tearing

MOUTH AND THROAT

Bad breath
Blisters, ulcers
Coated tongue
Dry mouth

Rash
Sore and bleeding gums
Sore and dry throat
White patches

SKIN

Acne
Athletes foot
Dermatitis
Dry scalp
Fungal infections of skin and nails

Itching
Psoriasis
Rashes
Skin discolouration

MUSCULAR SKELETAL SYSTEM

Arthritis
Joint pains
Joint stiffness
Joint swelling

Low back pain
Muscle aches and pains
Muscle paralysis
Muscle weakness

NOSE AND SINUSES

Itching
Nasal congestion and stuffiness

Post nasal drip

LUNGS AND CHEST

Asthma
Pain and tightness
Persistent cough

Shortness of breath
Wheezing

URINARY SYSTEM

Burning on urination
Cystitis *
Recurring bladder infections
Recurring kidney infections

Urethritis *
Urgency to urinate
Urinary infections

CARDIOVASCULAR SYSTEM

Cold hands and feet
Lack of libido *
Mitral valve prolapse
Palpitations

Poor circulation
Sexual impotence
Tingling and numbness in
extremities

EMOTIONAL / MENTAL NERVOUS SYSTEM

Acute anxiety
Agitation
Constant sleepiness
Depression
Extreme mood changes
Fatigue
Inability to concentrate
Irritability

Jittery behaviour
Lethargy
Nervous exhaustion
Panic attacks
Persistent headaches
Poor memory
Sudden mood swings

MISCELLANEOUS
Bad dreams
Dizziness
Hair loss
Increased body hair
Insomnia
Loss of appetite
Loss of balance

Loss of body hair
Overreacting
Poor co-ordination
Thyroid imbalances
Weight gain
Weight loss

WOMEN
Endometriosis
Extremely heavy menstrual flow
Failure to menstruate
Menstrual cramps
Non cancerous lumps in breasts
Premenstrual depression

Premenstrual tension
Scant menstrual flow
Soreness of breasts
Thrush
Too frequent periods

MEN
Prostatis *
Thrush under foreskin

ALLERGIC SYMPTOMS
Asthma
Food and chemical sensitivities
Hay fever

Hives
Rhinitis *
Urticaria *

Diseases thought to be related to, or affected by Candida albicans

A.I.D.S.
Alcoholism
Allergies
Anorexia nervosa
Autism
Bulimia
Cancer
Chrohn's disease
Chronic respiratory disease
Diabetes

Drug addiction
Epilepsy
Hodgkins disease
Inflammatory bowel disease
Multiple sclerosis
Myasthenia gravis
Sarcoidosis
Scleroderma
Systemic lupus erythematosus
Thyroid imbalances

M.E. sufferers will often have a history of what has been diagnosed as glandular fever and lymphatic glands will swell on a regular basis.

* For explanation of medical terminology see Glossary pages.

List of symptoms found in children with Candida albicans.

Chronic cough
Colic
Constipation
Craving for sweets
Diarrhoea
Digestive problems
Gas and bloating
Hyperactivity
Irritability
Learning difficulties

Mood swings
Nappy rash
Nasal congestion
Persistent headaches
Recurring ear infections
Short attention span
Thrush
Tonsillitis
Wheezing
Worm infestation

Children will also have a very 'pasty' grey complexion and often have dark rings under their eyes.

THANKS

One of the reasons this book came into existence is because so many people said "Thank you." They were grateful for the improvement in their health and lifestyle, and encouraged me to write down the advice I had given to them in order for others to benefit from it.

A word of thanks can be an inspiration. It can fire a person with enthusiasm and urge them on to better things. Whether we are paid for it, or are volunteers, we all work better when we know we are appreciated.

I now want to convey my thanks to all those who have been my clients and who have supplied me with the incentive to continue my work, sometimes in the face of stiff opposition. Also for all the letters they wrote, not only have they been an encouragement to me, but they have helped others who read them, to have hope

Also I owe thanks to all those who have helped and supported me in the writing of this book. I shall not mention names for fear of leaving someone out, they know who they are and are humble enough not to require public acclaim.

The only one who isn't going to be allowed to fade into the background as usual is my much appreciated, long suffering husband and partner, Ben. He tolerated the perpetual tap of the typewriter, corrected my spelling, edited and re-edited, did the typesetting and generated an atmosphere of peace, calm and love whilst we worked together. What a man! Thank you my love!

As you read, perhaps you can think of someone who has helped you in some way. Why not let them know how grateful you are.

"Go on, say thank you"

THRUSH

Thrush is the bane of some women's lives. In the clinic, women come for the first time and relate horrendous stories of how they have suffered this problem for most of their lives. Some starting in childhood. It can reduce a strong person to a quivering heap. The smallest dose of antibiotic will cause it to flare up, causing unbearable irritation and stripping the skin from the vagina and vulva. It often renders a woman incapable of sitting comfortably or walking and of course intercourse becomes impossible. What can be done to alleviate the problem.

In most cases, it must be understood to be an internal problem originating in the colon and working its way from the anus into the vagina. Think what a short distance it is and you will see how easily the yeast can migrate. If the problem is from colonic infestation then it will not be fully resolved until the colon is completely clear.

Much of this is caused by wearing clothing that is too tight around the genital area. It would be a good idea to wear loose panties and stockings instead of tights. Also when using tissue after a bowel movement, use an upward, backward stroke thus avoiding further infection reaching the vagina.

Men can be carriers of the infection under the foreskin and infect sexual partners, so super cleanliness should be observed during and after sexual intercourse. Careful washing both before and after will help reduce chances of further infection. Use of condoms will also help.

Until the colonic problem is resolved, all you can do is seek relief using localized treatments A variety of ideas are to be found under the heading, "Ways of avoiding the use of drugs." There are also helpful hints on dealing with oral thrush and infestations under the foreskin. A great deal of sympathy is needed to help you endure this symptom until it can successfully be brought under control. Keep working on it and it will respond eventually.

"Thrush is for the birds"

URINE

Frequent urination is often a troublesome symptom for both Candida and M.E. sufferers. This means they rarely sleep throughout the night without waking up to go to the lavatory.

They often find traveling any distance is difficult because they need to 'go' so many times en route and toilets are not always easy to find in strange territory.

Try not to worry too much, it is usually one of the first symptoms to respond well to treatment, but until it begins to lessen, try not drinking too many fluids after 6pm (take your 2nd dose of probiotic an hour before your evening meal when your stomach is empty instead of last thing before bed). Avoiding the 8oz of fluid at night may make all the difference. Likewise, don't drink for several hours before setting out on a long journey.

Under this heading it would be good to mention that whilst you are taking Vitamin B2 your urine will be a strong yellow colour. This is natural and totally harmless.

"It's just a wee problem"

USEFUL ADDRESSES

Dulwich Health Society, 130 Gypsy Hill, London, SE19 1PL Tel 0208 6705883. www.dulwichhealth.co.uk. (Helpful in identifying and correcting electromagnetism & geopathic stress problems)

Earthdust Products. 13 Glenwood Gardens, Hope Corner Lane, Taunton, Somerset. TA2 7PA Tel & Fax 01823 351108 (This company distributes the products described in this book. Many are available only through this outlet and are specially formulated for Jo Hampton to her own specifications. World wide mail order available)

Foyles Book Shop, Charing Cross Road, London WC2H OEB. (If difficulty is found purchasing books mentioned, try here)

Hal Huggins, Diagnostic Centre, P.O. Box 2589, Colorado Springs, LiCO 80901 U.S.A. International Code then 719 473 4702. (To obtain Hal Huggins books order direct from this address)

Hyperactive Childrens Support Group (HCSGG). 71, Whyke Lane, Chichester, West Sussex, PO19 2LD. Tel 01243 551313

National Candida Society P.O. Box 151, Orpington, Kent, BR5 1UJ (Support)

Interaction Journal Action for M.E. & Chronic Fatigue. P.O. Box 1302, Wells, Somerset, BA5 2WE Tel 01749 670799 (Will supply info and facts sheets)

Dr. Jack Levenson, 221 Old Brompton Road, London SW5 0EA Tel 020 7370 0055 (To order Dr. Levensons book direct by post.)

Lifestyle Health Care Ltd, Centenary Business Park, Henley-on-Thames, Oxfordshire RG9 1DS Tel 01491 570000 Fax 01491 570001 (Supply dairy free, gluten free, wheat free foods, ask for catologue)

Wholistic Research Company, The Old Forge, Mill Green, Hatfield Herts, AL9 5NZ Tel 01707 262686 www.wholisticresearch.com. (Filter systems, kitchen appliances, etc. Contact for more information)

Heal Farm, Kings Nympton, Umberleigh, Devon EX37 9TB Tel 01769 574341 www.healfarm.co.uk (Suppliers of organically reared meat, delivered)

Soil Association, Bristol House, 40-56 Victoria Street, Bristol, BS1 6BY Tel 0117 9290661 (Hold lists of suppliers of organic produce throughout the country)

VEGETARIANISM

To eat meat or not to eat meat, that is the question! Whether it be nobler.... I do agree vegetarianism is the better way to eat for many valid reasons all testified to by others before me, but particularly in the wake of B.S.E. For those with Candida M.E. and allergies it can be of great value because meat stays in the gut for an average of 12 hours whilst vegetables take only 4 hours to pass through the digestive system. This means meat will slow down the rate that all other foods take to pass through the alimentary tract.

Vital energy is needed to complete the digestive process so a meat eater will be more tired than a vegetarian counterpart. Also during the time the food lays in the body it is giving time for fermentation to take place. For someone fighting a Candida overgrowth this is disastrous. The fermentation encourages fresh overgrowth.

If you can, be a vegetarian. If you already are, continue, but unless you are knowledgeable about the nutritional values of foods, and the way to make sure your diet includes enough proteins from vegetable sources, then don't change whilst you are ill. It is extremely important to keep your vitamin, mineral and trace element intake high until your health improves.

A sensible compromise for the present would be to change to eating only chicken and fish, and always remember to eat fruit before flesh, so that fermentation of the fruit is prevented by making sure it does not become trapped behind the proteins.

I would encourage everyone to learn how to change to vegetarianism safely, making sure of a really well balanced diet.

"Give us only vegetables to eat, and water to drink.".. At the end of 10 days they looked healthier and were better nourished than... others" Daniel 1 v 12-15

VISION

Like Martin Luther King, I too have a dream.....

Most of those involved in alternative and complementary therapies are forward looking people who care deeply about the welfare of others.

They are prepared to risk opposition from orthodox medicine and the establishment. It is a great shame but this is the case. We should all be working in harmony, for the ultimate benefit of sick people, no matter what their illness is. Patients should not be penalized by mockery or in a financial way for preferring non drug therapies.

Their bodies are in their custody, therefore they are the ones who will live or die from the consequences of medicaments prescribed. I dream of a day when all doctors will hold a list of complementary practitioners in their area, and be willing to refer a patient to a therapist able to relieve their symptoms and pain by alternative means, should the patient wish it. This would of course necessitate doctors being instructed in the value of alternatives, and what they are able to accomplish, as part of their basic training.

It has already begun. In Germany, France and the Netherlands. In Britain osteopathy and acupuncture have become fairly acceptable and aromatherapy is being used in hospitals and in care of the elderly. It is a small beginning, but I visualize a time when health care authorities world wide will be prepared to use resources on preventative treatments, rather than allowing drug companies to perpetuate illness by masking symptoms and creating new problems with side effects. My vision sees children being educated about nutrition in school. Health care should be as important a subject as money management.

Yes, my dream sees a world society in which people can benefit from the treatment of their choice, or where....

"No resident in the land will say", 'I am sick'"
Isaiah 33 v 24

VITAMINS - & Minerals for your Programme

Because good vitamins are expensive, people often try to do with less than the programme recommends, but this is false economy since each one has an important part to play in rebuilding your immune system.

Taking each one separately, I will explain exactly what they do, why they are necessary and how they interrelate. (Called the synergistic effect.)

1) Vitamin A as Beta Carotene

Beneficial in the treatment of acne, failing eyesight, emphysema, hypertension and works in conjunction with B complex, Vitamin C and Zinc. It stimulates and activates T cells. Useful in viral diseases Vitamin A has long been shown to protect humans from bacterial, fungal and parasitic infections. Taken as Beta Carotine, rather than in retinol forms it scores, as it may be taken in high doses without incurring toxicity, sometimes occurring during prolonged ingestion of retinol. In laboratory tests Vitamin A has proved invaluable in restoring immunity.

2) Vitamin E (d Alpha Tocopherol)

Valuable for Candida and M.E. as it helps the supply of oxygen to the body, giving more endurance. Protects against air pollution by working with Vitamin A. It alleviates fatigue, one of the major symptoms of both C.A. and M.E. AS a diuretic can lower blood pressure. Vitamin E protects the fat cell membranes from damage called peridoxation. Works with Selenium to protect from malignant growths.

3) Vitamin C.

Is a catalyst for all other vitamins and minerals. Apart from its well known effects on viral infections, it has been proved to enhance T cells immune function. Vitamin C increases the ability of white cells in the blood to surround and destroy invaders. It increases production of natural interferon and is necessary for proper thyroid function. It protects the body generally against viral, fungal and bacterial infection. Vitamin C is also involved in protection of adrenal gland cortisol, a hormone which protects from stress. The body is incapable of manufacturing its own Vitamin C so daily supplementation is necessary. It acts as a natural laxative to alleviate constipation. Also reduces the affects of many allergens and over a period of time aids in rebuilding resistance Decreases infection by 25% and cancers by 75% according to Dr. Linus Pauling (Nobel Prize Winner).

4) Vitamin B5 Pantothenic Acid (one of the B complex) or Calcium Pantothenate.
Stimulates the immune system. Has been adequately demonstrated as being capable of enhancing activity of natural killer cells in the body. It is necessary for antibody protection (another branch of the immune system) and is most helpful in reducing stress factors. Invaluable as part of a comprehensive immune booster.

5) Magnesum Gluconate
Necessary for Vitamin C and Calcium metabolism. Essential for effective nerve and musle function. Really powerful aid in fighting depression. Brings relief from digestive problems. Is involved in protein synthesis inside the cells.

6) Vitamin B1
All B vitamins are synergistic, which means they are more potent together than individually. B1 is known as the 'Morale Vitamin' because of its beneficial effects on the nervous system and mental attitude. It is a mild diuretic. Aids digestion, especially of carbohydrates. Keeps the nervous system and muscles functioning.

7) Vitamin B3 (nicotinamide) Part of the B complex.
A person who is deficient in B, B2 and B6, will not be able to produce niacin. A lack of niacin can bring about negative personality changes. B3 is necessary for healthy sexual activity, strong nervous system and brain function. It also alleviates gastrointestinal disturbances.

8) B2, (part of the B complex)
Is not stored in the body so needs supplementation on a daily basis. It promotes healthy skin, nails and hair. Benefits vision and alleviates eye fatigue. Helps fight stress and anxiety.

9) Vitamin B6 Pyridoxine

Is involved in many chemical reactions in the body cells, especially in the essential fatty acid reactions. B6, is one of the most common vitamin deficiencies along with folic acid. Deficiency causes more impairment of immune function than any other vitamin. Its benefits include, alleviating nausea, reducing muscle spasms, leg cramps, hand and extremity numbness. Also useful against P.M.S and works as a natural diuretic.

10) Inositol.

Another part of the B complex. Works in conjunction with choline to form lecithin. Promotes healthy hair, aids in prevention of hair loss. Helps skin problems. Has been invaluable in nourishing brain cells. Helps fight eczema and aids redistribution of body fat.

11) Choline

Works in conjunction with inositol to utilize body fat and cholesterol. Aids in sending nerve impulses, especially those used in formation of memory in the brain. Assists in memory loss. Helps eliminate poisons and drugs from the system, by aiding the liver.

12) P.A.B.A. (para amino benzoic acid)

Helps form folic acid and is important in utilization of protein. Assists assimilation of pantothenic acid (another of the B vitamins). Revitalizes skin. Helps restore growth, colour and health to hair.

13) Zinc

Protects immune system and supports T cells. When zinc intake is decreased the thymus atrophies. The reason why this happens is yet to be discovered. Zinc is important in hormone production. Too much zinc is as bad as too little, so careful monitoring of intake is essential. Helps prostate problems and impotence, restores poor libido. Can be useful in regulating menses. Zinc works best where Vitamin A and Calcium are present.

14) Biotin (Vitamin H)

Needed to synthesize ascorbic acid (vitamin C). It is essential for normal metabolism of fats and protein. Vital in the synthesizing of intestinal bacteria. Works with B2, B6 and Vitamin A in maintaining healthy skin. Eases muscle pains.

15) Folic Acid

Is involved in the formation of white blood cells and lymphocytes, the front line of the immune system. When folic acid is diminished, the growth of T cells is reduced, stunting immune growth, and antibody production occurs. Folic acid protects against intestinal parasites, gives healthy looking skin and acts as an analgesic for pain. It increases appetite and helps ward off anemia.

16) Vitamin B12

Essential in the formation and regeneration of red blood cells. Increases energy. Maintains nervous system. Relieves irritability, and improves concentration and memory.

17) Selenium

Interestingly, Candida albicans infection in animals has been related to selenium deficiency. It helps prevent body fats becoming rancid and protects the body from toxic minerals like lead, mercury and cadmium. It should always be taken in conjunction with Vitamin E as they work in harmony.

When you understand the individual properties of all the vitamins and minerals included in your supplement list, you will realize why they are so essential, both to relieve your symptoms, and also how they work to rebuild your defective immune system. To be effective, these supplements need to be taken over an extended period in the doses recommended. It is advisable to have your vitamin levels monitored every two months to check that you still need the recommended doses.

"Keep taking the tablets"

WATER

Whatever you do, don't drink it straight from the tap. This is very important advice as chlorine is added to tap water, and in many parts of the world it is strong enough to knock your socks off. The reason chlorine is added in such large amounts is to kill harmful bacteria. The problem for you is that it can't differentiate between the harmful, and the "friendly flora." Therefore it can destroy all the expensive probiotics you have been trying to build up in your system.

In some places well water is available, but in most cases you would need to buy bottled water, or a filter. There are several kinds of filters. A jug can be purchased which you fill straight from the tap. A renewable filter is fitted to the jug and the water goes through making it useable. This is a portable method making it possible to treat water wherever go, but you need to keep refilling, and it takes patience to wait for the water to trickle through.

You might choose to have a filter fitted under your sink, with a special tap beside the others. This proves very convenient but only treats water coming to the sink.

Another system is to have a filter fitted to the rising mains water pipe in your home. This method treats all the water in the house. You are then able to have water 'on tap' whenever and where ever you need it. Since you must use pure water for all your cooking needs, this is the best idea if you can afford it.

The last suggestion is very helpful for those with skin problems as it filters bath and shower water, as well as the water used for washing clothes. Itching and burning skin can improve dramatically within a few days of installation.

"Water is the 'stuff' of life"
so
"Drink pure H_2O where ever you go"

WAYS OF AVOIDING DRUGS

Since it is important to avoid using chemical preparations and antibiotics, you need to know what to use as alternatives to treat common ailments.

Acne, all spots and insect bites
Tea Tree oil applied directly to affected parts. (May need diluting.)

Alternatives to prescription antifungal drugs
Caprylic acid is by far the most effective, particularly when it is enteric coated to ensure time release in the intestines. However, a minority find it abrasive to the system for other health reasons. They can use Pau D'Arco, oregano, grape seed extract, olive leaf extract or tea tree oil (caution if ingested, must be diluted carefully).

Catarrh, Coughs, Colds and Bronchial Infections
Inhale with Friars Balsam (Benzoin essential oil), Olbas Oil or Tiger Balm (melted). Line a bowl with foil and add a few drops to 500ml (1pt) of boiling water. Cover your head with a towel and inhale the concentrated fumes. Your bowl is protected by the foil as the oils tend to cling. You can also use Olbas and eucalyptus oil on your pillows, hankies and night clothes. Tiger Balm on your chest at night will free breathing. An effective, sugar free cough mixture can be made up by an experienced aromatherapist using a zanthan gum and water base with eucalyptus, hyssop and peppermint essential oils.

Constipation.
Vitamin C can be used effectively to alleviate constipation by taking more than the recommended daily allowance of between 45 & 60mg. Raise the dosage daily until a comfortable bowel movement is achieved, then continue on that dose until regular movements are restored. Herbs to help are Cape Aloe, Senna, Cascara, Ginger and Barberry. Some herbalists supply a mixture containing all these.

Ear Ache.
Place 5 drops lavender oil in a 10ml dropper bottle, then fill to the top with almond oil. Shake well. Stand bottle in hot water until oil is warm,

then put a few drops in each ear. Wiggle the lobes to help it down and add a piece of cotton wool to keep it warm. Repeat morning and evening.

Fungal infections of skin and nails
Use Tea Tree oil. Massage well into affected parts. It will take several days to see improvement, but keep it up, it works.

Headaches
Massage the temples, back of the neck and shoulders. Sit or lie with cold compress on back of neck or forehead depending on site of pain. Alternating hot and cold compresses helps. A compress can be made by soaking a guest towel or flannel in cold water and folding to required size. Sometimes sleep does the trick. Also try rubbing the reflexes of your big toe. Some people find relief from Tiger Balm across the forehead.

Hormone Disturbances
Oil of fennel is useful for stimulating hormones, particularly to help increase breast milk production. It can also be useful for hormonal help during menopause. Use 2 drops of fennel oil to 35ml (2fl oz) of water. Make sure the oil is well distributed and drink back quickly. Agnus Castus is also very good for all kinds of hormonal disturbances and Wild Yam will stimulate production of natural progesterone. These two are available in capsule form.

H.R.T. alternative
Use a Wild Yam supplement and add the boron supplement and gluco-samine sulphate suggested under osteoporosis, plus Fish oil.

Influenza
Select the remedies from this list that most fit your symptoms and go to bed. Stay there until you feel better. Not only will you recover more quickly if you rest, but you will avoid infecting others. Olive leaf extract, taken in advance can protect you from it.

Itching and cracked skin
Pure almond oil gently massaged in. If the skin is inflamed or chapped use Zinc and Caster Oil cream, (the kind used for babies bottoms). Calendular cream is also helpful.

Loss of Appetite
Is often due to zinc deficiency. Raising the daily intake of zinc will make a difference, but do not continue taking zinc for long without professional supervision as it is possible to take too much.

Osteoporosis
A trace element called boron builds healthy bones and is available in a complex form. Add to this a daily fish oil supplement together with glucosamine sulphate (derived from shell, not sugar) for regular, quality protection. Particularly useful for those with a tendency to arthritis. (See my book, The Arthritis Cookbook and Drug free Treatment Plan.)

Pain
See separate heading "Pain" on page 135. White Willow as a natural herbal pain killer. Check with practitioner for restrictions.

Parasites
Artemesia Complex. Combination of Cloves, Black Walnut Tincture and Wormwood. Regular use of zapper.

Sleeplessness (insomnia)
First check your room for good ventilation, with no drafts. Next, the weight of bedclothes and height of pillows. See that your night clothes are comfortable. Make sure your body temperature is right. If you are cold, fill a hot water bottle, if too hot, remove some of the covers. Remove yourself from a 'snore zone' if your partner is prone. Camomile tea can relax you, and passiflora and valerian are known to be sopophoric.

Some people find that Kava Kava helps them. Taking extra calcium can be useful. If you can enlist aid, a back massage works wonders. If everything fails, get up and do something. You will soon become tired and then you can go back and try again. Meanwhile it is surprising what you can achieve when the house is quiet and you have no interruptions. Geopathic stress might be a cause if you are regularly failing to have proper sleep. To check this:- contact The Dulwich Health Society (See page heading Useful Addresses)

Sore Throat

Swirl 5 drops of lavender oil, Tea Tree oil or Propolis in a glass of warm water and gargle with it. Don't spit it out, let it trickle down the back of your throat. It will continue to fight infection from within.

Thrush (oral)

Garlic or Tea Tree oil. 1 teaspoonful swirled round every corner of the mouth. Penetrate every corner. Hold it as long as you can then swallow it. It will continue to work down through the alimentary tract.

Thrush (vaginal)

It will clear as internal treatment takes effect but until then relieve it by regular douching with comfrey tea, made by pouring 500ml (1pt) of boiling water over 3 teaspoonsful of dried comfrey. Leave to stand, both to cool to body heat and to steep. Pau D'Arco and Tee-He-Bo tea are also useful for douching. Use once daily and follow by inserting (1) an acidophilus based cream (if not available use live yogurt). (2) Inserting a tampon soaked in garlic oil during the day and a tea tree oil pessary at night.

Toothache

Either a whole clove or a piece of cotton wool soaked in oil of cloves held firmly over the offending tooth. See a dentist as soon as possible.

If you need help with other drug free treatments, don't be afraid to contact me, care of the publisher. I will help if I can.

WEIGHT

Weight problems are common among sufferers from allergies, M.E. and Candida. It is a source of real worry to them. Both overweight and underweight can be induced by the illnesses.

Let's look first at underweight. Many people who have serious allergic reactions to food become afraid to eat. Some with digestive problems cannot assimilate food, however much they eat. It simply passes through the system without giving nourishment. Others may have parasites who devour the food to sustain themselves, leaving the person devoid of nourishment. Whatever the cause, it must be investigated and measures taken to correct the downward trend. Weight loss can only be allowed to go so far before it becomes dangerous.

Being overweight can also have several causes. The first, overeating and lack of exercise can be easily remedied, but some overweight people are heartily sick of others assuming this is always the case. It is not. Extra weight can accumulate when the body stores waste instead of eliminating it. It can be due to glandular disturbances or retention of lymphatic fluid. It is sometimes genetic, but that's rare.

Be encouraged by the knowledge that both situations are often reversed within a few weeks of beginning the programme, if the rules are strictly kept. The initial weight loss can be anything between 1.80 kilos(8lbs) and 13 kilos (2 stone) then it may slow down, and nothing more happen for a couple of months. Lymphatic massage can then be of value to restart the process, although it may prove painful the first time because the flesh will be tender.

Watching calorie intake always helps, but your prime objective should be optimum health. As your health improves your weight will stabilize at the right weight for you as an individual.

"Just you 'weight' and see"

WORM and Parasite Infestation.

Poor immune defences weaken resistance to all kinds of parasites. Many people who work with, or keep animals are subject to invasion by the ascaris worm. This parasite though originating in the intestines, becomes particularly active in the lungs giving rise to bronchial difficulties and asthma attacks although it is frequently able to migrate elsewhere in the body.

Since travel to warmer countries for holidays has become more popular, two other common parasites are Giardia lamblia and amebae.

Humans are particularly prone to parasite attack and many of the most common illnesses are being linked to parasite invasion in the affected organs, but by far the most common parasite infestation apart from Candida is thread worms. It isn't pleasant, but it happens when the immune system is at a low ebb. The recognizable symptoms will be, itching around the anus, particularly at night, continuous hunger, and possibly, unaccountable weight loss.

If you think you may have them, then you should check, and be sure. You will need to pass a motion in a shallow receptacle. An old fashioned chamber pot is ideal, but a bowl will do. Then, distasteful as this may seem to you, you must inspect the faeces. Thread worms look just as they sound, like little white threads. Be sure to look quickly because they will retreat into the mass of faeces fast, to keep warm. If they are present, you will see them wriggling. Once you are certain you have them, obtain medication to clear them from your system.

An aromatherapy preparation can be mixed by a knowledgeable practitioner to avoid using chemicals. If this is not possible, then go to your local chemist, and confide in him. He will suggest something and make it up for you if necessary. Whatever happens, clear them out fast, because whilst they remain they will undermine your health, and progress. After using the treatment, check again to make sure you are clear, by using the 'potty procedure' described above.....and cheer up!

"It could happen to anyone"

XMAS

Every year, around the beginning of November, people who have been regularly attending the clinic and making excellent progress, phone to cancel their appointments or stop taking their supplements. They are saving up for Christmas...

They couldn't choose a worse time of year to let down their defences. In the Northern hemisphere it is the time when coughs, colds, 'flu' and infections of all descriptions are rampant. With a depressed immune system, they are an easy target. They catch them all.

Then comes *The Big Holiday.* Everyone around is stuffing themselves full of the worst kind of sweet, sugary, yeasty, milky, gooey foods. The silent sufferer watches in agony, drooling and fighting their conscience, then finally they weaken and indulge as a loving, kindly, friend or relative says, "Go on, just a little bit can't hurt." *But it does hurt,* particularly the next day when they can't get out of bed.

Before they know it, they are back to their original poor condition, with all the old familiar symptoms. By the first week in January, my appointment book is full to overflowing with those wanting me to work a miracle. Sorry, not possible. They'll have to start again. It's a long haul back over the ground that has been lost.

"Please, please, please! Don't do it"